T0285834

# MEDICAL POLITICS

# MEDICAL POLITICS

## HOW TO PROTECT YOURSELF FROM BAD DOCTORS, INSURANCE COMPANIES, AND BIG GOVERNMENT

## STEPHEN SOLOWAY, MD

### WITH DENISE LISTER, CMA
### FOREWORD BY SEAN WEISS

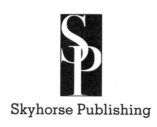

Skyhorse Publishing

In loving memory of my wonderful parents,
Frances and Warren Soloway

# WHAT PATIENTS HAVE TO SAY
# ABOUT DR. SOLOWAY

"I have known Dr. Soloway since 1977 when he moved to Great Neck and we went to high school together. I later heard that he was a doctor that treated joints. Years ago, I reached out to him for a problem with my wrist. I had already been to the 'best' hand doctors in New York and Long Island. They both wanted to operate.

I met with Dr. Soloway (I call him Steve) five years ago. He injected medicine at the base of my thumb where it meets the wrist. Overall, it was so successful I never went back to any surgeon and I do not understand why they did not offer this treatment nor why they would not refer me to a rheumatologist. Dr. Soloway's book is reminiscent of this true story. It is so true and so spot on. He describes all the pitfalls of the past ten to fifteen years, why they have occurred, and what solutions can be utilized. He points out that the government has forced us into socialized medicine and we are only noticing it now. This book is a must-read. I am so proud to know the author and call him a dear friend."

—Maria Mastramatteo

"I am a patient of Dr. Soloway's. I was placed in the hospital for a five-day period of time for severe abdominal pain and diagnosed with pancreatitis. I was discharged from the hospital with the same pain that got me admitted. I went to Dr. Soloway because of my abdominal pain and because I trust him so much. My sister has been affiliated with his office for her entire working career and she trusts him as well. She advised me to see him even though it was out of his field. He spoke to me for fifteen or thirty minutes, he examined me, and—this is what struck me when he pushed on my belly, he asked me if it hurt more when I push or when I let go. I answered his question. He then asked me how it compared to when I was in the hospital. I replied that nobody touched me when I was in the hospital at all. I was never examined. The CAT scan of my pancreas was normal, yet I was told I had pancreatitis.

Dr. Soloway was positive that I had both inflammatory bowel disease and associated arthritis. He started me on oral steroids and I was almost 100 percent better within twenty-four hours. After this episode he asked me to peruse his book. I did so gladly. I can say without a doubt and under no uncertain terms that the healthcare system is terrible and Dr. Soloway is able to sort it all out and to explain it to people in a way they will understand, especially by including letters that he wrote on behalf of patients to insurance companies. There is no reason why people are not referred properly and everybody should read this book because it is honest and truthful. I felt like I was reading about myself throughout the whole book. And by the way my hospitalization cost more than $40,000 while I wasted away. Dr. Soloway got probably less than $200, and he was able to make the correct diagnosis."

—Regina Hester

"As a patient of Dr. Soloway's, I would never complain about his waiting time. I relish that I was fortunate enough to see him. For fifteen years I suffered abdominal pain, joint pain, abdominal cramps, and passing blood. During one visit with Dr. Soloway, he looked at an x-ray of my sacroiliac joint that he did in the office and he told me that I had either Crohn's disease or ulcerative colitis. I needed a biopsy, but the initial treatment would be the same. I had a biopsy which showed I have Crohn's disease. With his treatment I was 100 percent better in a very short time. Fifteen years of suffering had ended.

Six months after I started treatment and had a normal life, my insurance company denied my medication. This book addresses situations like mine and probably yours. I have seen how Dr. Soloway's job has become nothing but fighting for patients and screaming at insurance companies and I can honestly say you must read this book."

—Mario Marcucci

# CONTENTS

# FOREWORD
# The Landscape of Healthcare
## SEAN WEISS

My introduction to Stephen Soloway, MD, was typical in my line of work: payers were auditing and demanding money back from his rheumatology practice in New Jersey, and he had enough! My firm has engaged in a number of payer issues both on the government and commercial payer side and had success in getting payers to back down or close their investigations. Stephen's story of ongoing harassment by payers would have been just another of hundreds of thousands of stories, but he has been fighting back, forcing payers to make decisions in his favor that they otherwise would not have made.

When I was first asked to write the foreword to this book, I was caught by surprise. But as I listened to Dr. Soloway—"Doc," as I like to refer to him—I realized that not only did I have to, but also it became my mission. Physicians all over the country just like Stephen are fed up with the government's, their contractors', and commercial payers' unethical business practices but struggle with how to fight back. This book is a roadmap for health-care providers and health-care professionals to utilize lessons learned for you and your organization.

If you don't consider healthcare to be political, you should—and by the end of this book, you will. Politics has been playing a heavy role in health-care, because it is a $3.65 trillion industry (approximately 18 percent of the USA GDP[1])! Approximately 784,000 companies are in the health-care space,

---

1  Smilijanic Stasha, "The State of the Healthcare Industry—Statistics for 2022," Policy Advice (website), March 5, 2022, https://policyadvice.net/insurance/insights/health care-statistics/.

with McKesson being the largest by revenue at $208.3 billion. One of the biggest problems we face, if not the biggest, is that costs for healthcare are two times higher in the United States than anywhere else in the world. Yet, sadly, we rank eleventh in the world in performance (access to care, care process, administrative efficiency, equality, and health-care outcomes), which falls well below other countries such as Switzerland and Canada.[2] However, the landscape of healthcare is dynamic and continuously evolving (or regressing, depending on where you sit and your role as a health-care professional). Healthcare will play a key role in the 2024 presidential election, right behind inflation and border security.

The health emergency of the pandemic exposed the many failures of leadership at health systems, of elected officials, and of those responsible for the supply chain, resulting in catastrophic failures and unnecessary death for so many. More and more Americans are recognizing the ride we have been taken on by corporations that reaped some of the highest profits ever, as government has increased the sustainability of Social Security and the Medicare trust fund well beyond initial expectations. This is based largely on the amount of money coming back into the system from recoveries, court verdicts, and settlement agreements.

Members of our government who were put in place to protect us boldly lied to Congress and the American people about many things, including, but not limited to, the number of COVID-19-related deaths, whether masks protect us, the actual origins of the virus, and having enough tests, including at-home rapid tests. We dealt with a virus (with twenty-plus variants) that was more adaptable than the politicians elected by the people, for the people! The first year of the Biden White House and a Democratic-led Congress showed inconsistencies and failure in policy! This is not a partisan shot but a statement based on the administration's and Democrats' own

---

2    Eric C. Schneider et al., "Mirror, Mirror, 2021: Reflecting Poorly," The Commonwealth Fund, August 4, 2021, https://www.commonwealthfund.org/publications/fund-reports/2021/aug/mirror-mirror-2021-reflecting-poorly.

acknowledgment of failure. Policies on boosters, at-home testing, masking, and quarantines made the country's Omicron wave far worse than it should have been. The Centers for Disease Control and Prevention (CDC), Food and Drug Administration (FDA), and National Institutes of Health were slow to respond and inconsistent with their messaging and, in several instances, went against generally accepted standards of medical care to continue pushing forward political narratives for their boss on Pennsylvania Avenue! Congressional hearings have exposed the deception and, in many cases, the cover-up of incompetence.

Many politicians used the pandemic to grab political power and to politicize the health system to a level not seen before. Executive orders and false narratives led to our country teetering on the brink of recession. Inflation accelerated by 7.5 percent between January 2020 and January 2021, a forty-year high, as gas prices soared across the country, with oil crossing the $100-per-barrel threshold at times. Paychecks have been eroded by 1.7 percent since 2021, and the Medicare Part B premium increase our seniors were hit with is the largest in history. Going to the grocery store costs consumers close to $1,000 per month more than what they had been paying for decades—that's more painful than going to the proctologist! In July 2020 the inflation was reported at 9.1 percent, far beyond what the Biden Administration, including Janet Yellen of the Federal Reserve, believed it would be, further crushing American families and businesses.

President Biden blamed the failures of his administration on Trump, Trump supporters, COVID-19, and the Saudi Crown Prince (who was referred to as leading a pariah state, but then in July Biden went on bended knee asking for increases in oil production) until members of his own party and those in mainstream media who supported him, and the Democratic party, turned on him. Then came the Russian invasion of Ukraine, a new convenient situation to blame for a complete and utter failure of this administration. Government is inefficient and incapable of doing things well, which is why the private sector in healthcare is so critical to sustainability and advancements in treatments.

But Biden and his administration were only just beginning to wreak havoc on the health-care industry. All the Trump-era policies that reduced the regulatory burden on providers and the industry were erased with the stroke of a pen, creating what can only be described as the new era in healthcare.

Think about this: In fiscal year (FY) 2021, the government recouped from providers more than $1.8 billion, and it wasn't just from hospitals or health systems:

> In FY 2021, the Department of Justice (DOJ) opened 831 new criminal healthcare fraud investigations. Federal prosecutors filed criminal charges in 462 cases involving 741 defendants. A total of 312 defendants were convicted of healthcare fraud related crimes during the year. Also, in FY 2021, DOJ opened 805 new civil healthcare fraud investigations and had 1,432 civil healthcare fraud matters pending at the end of the fiscal year. Federal Bureau of Investigation (FBI) investigative efforts resulted in over 559 operational disruptions of criminal fraud organizations and the dismantlement of the criminal hierarchy of more than 107 healthcare fraud criminal enterprises.

It didn't stop there:

> In FY 2021, investigations conducted by HHS's Office of Inspector General (HHS-OIG) resulted in 504 criminal actions against individuals or entities that engaged in crimes related to Medicare and Medicaid, and 669 civil actions, which include false claims and unjust-enrichment lawsuits filed in federal district court, and civil monetary penalty (CMP) settlements. HHS-OIG also excluded 1,689 individuals and entities from participation in Medicare, Medicaid, and other federal healthcare programs. Among these were exclusions based on criminal convictions for

crimes related to Medicare and Medicaid (569) or to other health-care programs (267), for beneficiary abuse or neglect (145), and as a result of state healthcare licensure revocations (536).[3]

Recently, I was the expert in one of the largest health-care fraud trials, *United States of America v. D-1 Rajendra Bothra, D-4 David Lewis, and D-5 Christopher Russo.* The defendants were charged with fifty-four counts of violation of the Substance Control Act and the HealthCare Fraud Statute, for $484 million. One of the defendants (Bothra) spent three and a half years in federal detention and was denied bail and compassionate release nine times, while the others were basically put out of business and bankrupted. At the end of the trial, he and the other three defendants were found not guilty on all counts. Something like this can happen to anyone, anywhere, and at any time. This was a total political hack on the part of the government, so much so that one of the prosecutors resigned on the last day of the trial. I hope providers and health-care professionals will take proactive steps to mitigate risk and realize that no one is immune to aggressive investigations and over-zealous prosecutions.

Every administration has had missteps and missed opportunities to fix the health-care system, but all made empty promises, whether it was President Clinton failing to sign the Patient Bill of Rights; President George W. Bush failing to address the problem of millions of uninsured Americans and the rising costs of healthcare, refusing to expand eligibility for the state Children's Health Insurance Program (CHIP), taking maneuvers to cut Medicaid spending, or making unjustified subsidies for private health plans; President Obama enacting the Affordable Care Act (ACA) and forc-ing providers on to Electronic Medical Records (EMR); or Trump failing to repeal and replace ACA. Some were influenced by corporate money, whereas others were just incompetent in the health-care space because

---

3    Department of Health and Human Services and Department of Justice HealthCare Fraud and Abuse Control Program, *Annual Report for Fiscal Year 2021*, 2022,

they aligned themselves with equally incompetent yes people. Although all of the aforementioned presidents most likely had good intentions regarding how to fix the health-care system, no matter what they did, it would simply not be enough given the state of the industry and the level of corruption.

Overzealous and inexperienced prosecutors at the Department of Justice (DOJ) are aggressively pursuing providers in the name of integrity of the Medicare Trust Fund. The Office of Inspector General (OIG) predicts $3 billion in recoveries in FY 2022, which will drastically exceed FY 2021, from a variety of providers, including hospitals, nursing homes, infusion centers, physician practices and physician groups, ambulatory surgery centers, pharmacies, and suppliers.

*Azar vs. Allina Health Systems* (a 2019 Supreme Court ruling) pushed back on the Centers for Medicare and Medicaid Services for making substantive changes to policies not put through the formal rule-making process. However, the DOJ and OIG continue to rely on subregulatory documents as opposed to following regulations and pushing the envelope to see to what extent they can get away with fleecing the U.S. Health System.

Bounty hunters—Recovery Audit Contractors (RACs), Maximum Allowable Charges (MACs), Unified Program Integrity Contractors (UPICs)—of the government are incentivized to take aggressive positions against providers of health-care services because they are shielded from liability by the Centers for Medicare and Medicaid Services (CMS). They make determinations that adversely affect physicians' ability to render care to their patients. One might call the processes witch hunts. These contractors typically have five-year terms; if they fail to demonstrate return on investment, their contracts might not be renewed, so taking overzealous positions on audits or investigations should be expected by providers of medical care. Commercial insurance companies such as UnitedHealthcare, Blue Cross Blue Shield, Aetna, and Humana continue to cut provider reimbursement and patient access to care (testing, procedures, medications), all in the name of profit.

As a subject-matter expert who consults and testifies in a number federal civil and criminal health-care cases each year and testifies in dozens of administrative proceedings, I can share with you firsthand accounts of the dysfunction of the system and the uneven playing field. I have testified in cases in which the prosecutor read from a Medicare manual, not realizing that section failed to apply to the type of entity being prosecuted. I am constantly engaged in negotiations between providers and the Office of Inspector General, which in the last year seems to have lost its willingness to engage in good-faith negotiations and instead takes aggressive, over-the-top positions to try to force a settlement since it knows litigating a $150,000 case is simply not feasible. Insurance companies expect providers to render services without the companies paying them or paying them accurately or paying them in a timely manner. Some government and commercial payers place providers on 100 percent prepayment review, which leads either to delayed payment or no payment at all, but they expect providers to render services and expend costs with great financial risk. I have had payers say on calls, "Contractually, you have to see and treat our patients," to which we respond, "And you have to pay the claims. When you have paid the claims correctly and timely, we will again see and treat your members."

It's Business 101: you cannot continue to spend money and render services for free and expect to have a sustainable business model! Ultimately, you have to stand your ground with payers to not only sustain but also thrive in this industry.

At the end of this year, 2022, I will have dedicated twenty-eight years to the health-care industry. I have been blessed to have a career that I truly enjoy and have given my very best to. I have been honored throughout my career with awards, accolades, and recognition. I've engaged with members of Congress in both the upper and lower chambers, worked for the Department of Defense in Europe at both Landstuhl and Ramstein air bases, interviewed some of the most influential and important people in our industry, published in the industry's most authoritative sources, served on a governor's task force, and lectured at some of the most prestigious institutions in this great country of ours. But the most important thing I accomplished over my career was to create lifelong friendships with some of the most amazing and interesting people. Stephen Soloway is not only an interesting person but also quite possibly the most interesting man I have ever known. After reading *Bad Medicine*, Stephen's first book, I kept thinking, *There has to be a sequel!* Well, here it is, and I could not be more excited about it!

# INTRODUCTION:
# RAW TRUTH

What follows is the truth of medical politics—raw, unfiltered, appalling, deplorable, corrupt, disgraceful, disgusting, surprising, shocking—and every word of it is true. In short, the politics of medicine is such that if you are a patient and you don't fight, you will not get treated. And if you are a doctor and you aren't fighting, you are not doing your job.

Make no mistake: the government, the insurance companies, and the drug companies want it this way. They do not want you to know that you have power in this system. They want you to go back to your family doctor, and they want that doctor to say, "Here's some Percocet; you'll be fine."

The medical system is deeply broken. But a backstory tells the truth. The public may not know it; even I only know the half of it. But I'm not afraid to ask questions and write about what I see every day in my practice. Hold on—it's shocking.

Who am I? I'm Dr. Stephen Soloway, and, simply put, I'm the self-proclaimed best combination rheumatologic and orthopedic doctor alive. I've been named one of America's Top Doctors by *U.S. News & World Report* more times than anyone. I've been appointed by President Trump to the President's Council on Sports, Fitness & Nutrition, and Governor Chris Christie appointed me to the New Jersey Board of Medical Examiners. I am the division chief of rheumatology at the Inspira Health Network, where I designed the curriculum for my field. I've treated more billionaires, professional athletes, celebrities, and dignitaries than I can name. I've been practicing medicine for over thirty years, and I've seen absolutely everything. I've seen things in healthcare that would make the average American sick. I wrote an entire book about the horrors of American healthcare.

This is a book about politics—about bad government, bad hospitals, bad drug companies and insurance companies, and bad doctors. It's all connected, and at the very bottom, it's the patient—you!—who is getting screwed.

Take the hospitals: the hospital employs all the doctors these days. Those doctors are given a fifteen-minute slot to evaluate, treat, and document all the information they can get from a patient. They're not able to do a physical exam, so they just order a CT scan of anything and everything and hope that that will give them an answer. Sometimes it helps. Other times it's confusing because it will show red herrings.

But the pressure is on the doctor, and the doctor, in haste, just does something to appease somebody. Many of these doctors are undertrained and afraid to think outside the box. Guess who suffers? That's right—the patient.

Unless you are a cash-paying patient and you find a superstar doctor, you don't really count in this system. Most people who take chronic narcotics are either self-treating depression or another mental illness, or they were an addictive personality. But if you ask them what hurts, since they don't really know, they just say everything hurts.

People don't know what a rheumatologist is or does. Even the American College of Rheumatology doesn't know what a rheumatologist is supposed to do. You should not have to be a superstar to cover all the aspects of the field. You should be able to competently diagnose and treat rheumatoid arthritis, lupus, psoriatic arthritis, vasculitis, myositis, and scleroderma. In addition, you should be an expert in injecting trigger fingers, all tendons and bursae, arthritic thumbs, tennis elbow, rotator cuff, plantar fascia, Achilles tendons, low-back facet joints, knees, shoulders, hips, hands, and wrists, and maybe injecting epidurals, which I don't do. But I do lumbar facet and cervical facetted injections. Simply stated, for every field of orthopedics—hand surgery, back surgery, knee surgery, shoulder surgery, and so on—a good rheumatologist will always perform better. I can't see everyone. Lord knows I try!

Because I'm the only rheumatologist on the planet who's proficient in this degree in these injections at this time, I look like a criminal to people (such as those in the bureaucracy) who don't understand a very simple fact: I work hard. If you compare me to orthopedics and to pain management, I may still be up at the top of the list, but I wouldn't be alone. So I stand out— brightly—and nobody can understand how one person can be so effective, efficient, smart, and *not* be stealing.

A rheumatologist must be an amazing interrogator. You must drag the information from the patient. If you know what to ask and how to extrapolate information, you will get the answers. If you get the answers to the right question, you will know what's wrong 95 percent of the time, before you ever touch the person, before you even order the blood test. A rheumatologist should also be a gentle, precise injection expert.

Once, a woman was referred to me for a supposed diagnosis of rheumatoid arthritis. Right off the bat, I asked, "Ma'am, why did you have the rheumatoid factor drawn in the first place?"

"I don't know," she said. "That's part of the routine blood work?"

It isn't. Therefore, my index of suspicion immediately goes down because she didn't say it was ordered for joint pain or morning stiffness. "Why did you go to the doctor?" I asked.

"Well, after I was treated for my breast cancer, I had follow-ups."

"Oh, you had breast cancer? What type of breast cancer did you have? Was it estrogen-receptor positive, progesterone-receptor positive, or HER2 positive? Which breast cancer did you have?"

"I don't know."

"What do you mean?"

"Well, the lymph node biopsy didn't say."

"Well, what did the breast biopsy show?"

"I never had one."

"What do you mean?"

"Well, they couldn't really find anything. So they did a lymph node biopsy."

I asked if she has dry eyes.

She said, "Yes. Severely dry eyes and dry mouth. In fact, I have an erosion in one eye. And my mouth is drying. I'm losing my teeth."

I replied, "I need to see the biopsy report as to your breast-cancer diagnosis."

I did some blood, brought the person back, diagnosed her with Sjogren syndrome, and predicted that she had a lymphoma and never had breast cancer. I was right. Now, to get this person treated for lymphoma, she had to go on a whole other round of medicine, but she wouldn't because she maxed out the lifetime dose of whatever the particular chemotherapy agent was that she took. She ended up dying due to lymphoma, which briefly went into remission from the breast cancer protocol then came out of remission.

The patient should have seen a good rheumatologist much earlier. I see totally preventable tragedies like this all the time, and it makes me crazy.

Of course, there is a shortage of rheumatologists (which is fine because it makes me busier!). Not only is there a shortage, but also people don't even know why they should be using us in the first place. The local teaching hospital just took the rheumatology elective off the criteria of the core curriculum.

People say, "Rheumatologists . . . what do they do, exactly?" You'll hear it from politicians, janitors, educated authors, educated writers, and doctors of all fields.

The rheumatologist is the general contractor. He farms out if he needs a subcontractor. If you need a bone fixed, the rheumatologist calls the carpenter—that's your orthopedic doctor. If you need a nerve biopsy or spine surgery, he or she calls your neurosurgeon. It should all go through the rheumatologist.

Today, trainees are dictated to (or brainwashed) to be general practitioners (GP) or hospitalists or are told that they can be a nine-to-four, four-days-a-week rheumatologist and just triage patients. Sadly, the teaching hospitals tell the doctors to work for the system, as they will make more money. (What a load of rubbish that is.) I say work for yourself, not a system. The system will always rip you off. (Warren Buffet is credited with this phrase, but I was saying it before I knew who Buffet was.)

In most cases, it is cheaper to train and hire a nurse practitioner or physician assistant. But there is some hope. Take Audrey, for example. At approximately twenty-four years of age, Audrey graduated from an Ivy League nursing program in which she was granted a free ride due to her athletic ability. When she first joined me, the conversation started in my typical fashion—very aggressive and pushy. I told her on the phone, "Please come today for an interview. I need to hire you."

She replied, "I'm going on my honeymoon."

"You can go on your honeymoon any time! The job is more important," I responded.

She ended up going on her honeymoon. I called her the day she got back and said, "I need you to come down for your interview today."

She said, "I can't. I have to check with my husband."

"Who cares?" I said. "You are on the phone with me! It's something you have to decide, and your husband should have little to say about this job or your career."

When she finally came down, I said, "OK, you can start today." For various reasons, she couldn't start that day. But she started soon after, and within two weeks I'd given her the lay of the land. I explained all the bad medicine—everything from the uneducated and unqualified to just basic misfits in society that landed in our region. She admittedly found everything I said baffling and confusing and probably thought I was a blatant liar.

Six months later we were best friends, and we remained best friends until she had to relocate twelve years later. Within three months of working with me, she would tell anyone that everything that came out of my mouth was true no matter how crazy it sounded or how much it seemed like an exaggeration. Anything I told her that she failed to believe she had then seen with her own eyes—all the horrors that nobody else will talk about, that everyone—everyone—turns their back on. Imagine: ten gout patients on rheumatoid arthritis meds and ten rheumatoid arthritis patients on gout meds. Think I'm not serious? Think again.

She went on to run a rheumatology practice in another state and educate four rheumatologists with less knowledge than she had regarding disease recognition or injection techniques and other skills required of a rheumatologist. They were astounded by her injection skills and didn't understand how she knew so much. (They had never heard of me.)

Here is her story, in her own words:

I went to the University of Pennsylvania for my undergraduate degree, and I have two master's degrees in adult health and Gerontology from the University of Pennsylvania as well.

Dr. Soloway sent a request for an ad through the University of Pennsylvania School of Nursing. I responded to the email, and that's how we got connected.

When I started there, I was a new grad out of grad school. I was fairly naive as far as how the real world works. The biggest challenge was that Dr. Soloway's office was extremely fast-paced. But he was great because he let me in on the business side of things.

What was shocking was understanding the world of commercial insurance.

I never believed anything he said until I saw it for myself. When he would tell me these things over the phone, before I started working there or before I encountered it, I thought he had to be lying or over-exaggerating. There was no way. This is not really happening. Then I realized, "Oh, okay. It's true, all of it."

It was difficult and time-consuming to realize that much of your patient care can be dictated by their insurance company, as far as who they can see, where they can go, how quickly they can get in, what drugs they can have, what they have to go through before they are able to have that drug. Unless you have the support staff like Dr. Soloway does, it's almost impossible to function as a private practice nowadays, because you cannot do what you love, which is the clinical care, if you have to spend the majority of your day on the phone, supposedly speaking to a peer (never a true peer) to get something approved. There are only so many hours in the day. And most practices don't build in any administration time, whether that's for charting or billing or any phone calls or communication with anyone. So you don't have that time to get on the phone with an insurance company. You could spend an hour easily just hitting the prompts to get someone on the phone.

One of my professors was the very famous H. Ralph Schumacher Jr., MD, who literally wrote the book on synovial fluid and more. We learned back then that, in rheumatology, if you see fluid and you don't drain it, you are fired—you are an idiot; you don't belong. At one point, the *New England Journal of Medicine* solicited Ralph Schumacher to write an article on monoarthritis. He passed it off to one of his staff, Dan Baker, and Dan wrote the article.

I was there when the *New England Journal* called to say it couldn't accept it.

"Why not?"

"It says all joint effusions need to be tapped."

"They do," he said.

"Well, if you write that, then you are going to create chaos in the community."

Ah ha! So you are not allowed to write the truth. Well, I'll do it anyway.

How's this for the truth? The entrepreneurial private practitioner is a dying breed in medicine.

Having hospitals own the practices is a simple way to regulate hospitals, rather than having to regulate doctors. Regulating one hundred or one thousand hospitals is a lot easier than regulating a million individual doctors. That's all it's about. Your doctor is criminalized and penalized if he or she is perceived as being too busy.

When Trump was president, I met with the head of fraud and abuse at Medicare. I had to tell this person the history of Medicare fraud and abuse, to broaden the views of who and how people should be targeted. I had to explain *to her* what she should actually be looking for from an insider's standpoint. She didn't give a fuck.

This is what you get when you have Communists running the country and two political classes: the billionaires and the peasants. If you are not a billionaire, sorry, you are a peasant. We're all peasants because we don't have any control.

While we have no control, the government is out to destroy businesses as quickly as it can. Antiquated laws that benefit the government never seem to go away. An example would be wearing a mask. You still have to wear a mask in my office. Why? Who the hell knows? Most are vaccinated, and frankly, if you are not vaccinated by now, you should either know you are going to die, maybe, and it's up to you. Anyone that doesn't believe in the vaccine, I believe, is part of the problem. It's about control.

You must think outside the box. I'm the only guy I know that thinks outside the box. Why? Because not everything is in the box!

# CHAPTER 1
# MEDICAL ETHICS (NOT!)

## Nothing Is Ethical

Nothing in medicine is ethical—nothing. I've seen things in healthcare that most people would not believe—corruption, negligence, malpractice, stupidity, bureaucracy, theft, dishonesty, fraud, deception. You name it, I've seen it. Why? Because unethical behavior is ubiquitous, common knowledge, and not only tolerated but encouraged!

Ethics is ambiguous. Doctors are stuck between rules and proper patient management. Following the rules may disallow correct treatment, whereas white lies ("fraud," per the FBI, OIG, etc.) get patients a higher chance of better care. I don't treat colds; my patients are often deathly ill. If I did not fight for them, they would be dead. Gilding the lily can be easy as there are no peer-to-peer reviews. I have never once spoken to an actual peer!

Doctors can be unethical, but far more often it's the system—the hospitals, the government, the pharmaceutical companies, and the insurance companies—that is the real problem. With so much overreach, overregulation, and overadministration, the system has created an environment where doctors feel they *need* to be sneaky to do their job and hospitals feel free to screw patients left and right.

A doctor sometimes has to list the wrong diagnosis just to get a medicine approved because the insurance companies will not approve the medicine for anything other than the disease it was studied for. For example, I know from decades of experience that Remicade works for arthritis and ten other afflictions. But unless a person has *rheumatoid arthritis*, the insurance denies it. "Sorry," the company representative says, "there is no data." When

I send the person nine articles showing that it works, I hear that those weren't clinical trials, and they don't really count. So I have no choice but to modify the diagnosis. My responsibility as a physician is to get people the medicine they need. Is it unethical of me? Maybe, but what choice do I have in this system? The important thing is that the patient receives the necessary treatment, but the lengths a good doctor has to go to in this environment are extraordinary.

Then there is the hospital administrator. A hospital administrator will go to the ER and say, "admit all people who come in tonight, no matter what's wrong with them." They will then fudge the charts to make people look sicker. They will keep people alive on a ventilator (if their insurance is good) just to bill for ICU days. Filled beds equate to more money! (If the insurance is lousy, sometimes they'll simply euthanize.)

It's a travesty of medicine. And it is always—always—the patients who suffer.

It's a setup, a scam—fake work. Because at the same time that hospitals are ruining healthcare, the government is pushing to have hospitals run everything, because of ease of regulation I discussed earlier. Therefore, hospitals are not subjected to the kinds of audits that private practitioners like me are subjected to. Rarely will a hospital get audited, and when it is the hospital will not even get a slap on the wrist.

You will *not* see places like the University of Pennsylvania, Thomas Jefferson Cooper University, Drexel, Robert Wood Johnson, Johns Hopkins, or NYU subjected to the kind of onerous, oppressive, tyrannical, idiotic audits that I am subjected to on a routine basis.

The hospitals are protected because of donations or grants, which is how the deeply unethical system of bartering works at that level. Of course, it's also the reason that medical care is so bad at the top institutions. The top doctor at the top institution is getting his or her money by researching one disease and writing proposals for money in order to get the experimental or nonexperimental, nonapproved drugs. If the hospital can participate in that kind of trial, it gets a huge amount of money, which keeps its researchers busy not seeing patients and not teaching too much. All of this comes at the cost of taking care of patients.

Furthermore, in the hospital, doctors are paid by relative value units (RVUs). If you stay on time and don't spend more than fifteen minutes with a patient, including time spent at the computer, the hospital is happy with you. If you are providing good care and running late as a result, you get yelled at and reprimanded. So across the board, people in the hospitals are not doing their jobs because it's easier and less perilous to simply fly under the radar. It's not because they are dumb either. They're smart; they're sneaking through an unethical system and exploiting it.

All the while, the patient continues to suffer and the institution wins, ethics be damned. The only way to break this cycle is to encourage and incentivize people to be more entrepreneurial, to have the spirit of being self-employed. When you are self-employed, you really *do* care a lot more. You are not running out the door at 4:45. You just want to help your patients. You do not care about the hospital, the administrator, or the institution at large. If you are self-employed and helping your patients, you are helping yourself. It's a simple equation.

The hospital only looks out for itself. Not long ago, I received the following email from the University of Pennsylvania's Rheumatology Department:

> The *U.S. News & World Report*—Best Hospitals. Vote soon!
>
> Have you voted?
>
> Please join your peers in casting a vote for the Hospitals of the University of Pennsylvania-Penn Presbyterian among your nominations for best rheumatology care.
>
> VOTE NOW!
>
> Including a vote for Penn Medicine reinforces the reputation of the Penn Rheumatology community.

Now, you might say, "What's the big deal? It looks like a harmless letter." It is a big deal because it's illustrative of the unethical ways in which hospitals work—or, more accurately, don't work at all. The email had no purpose other than to tell everyone to vote for the hospitals of University of Pennsylvania on the *U.S. News and World Report*. The hospital is browbeating people to vote for it. I didn't get a letter from any other hospital. What's the problem? There is no doctor at Penn who is as good as I am—no one, and it's not even close. The other problem—soliciting votes for the title of "best"? Are you fucking kidding me?

It's consumer marketing to people that are mostly very stupid. It's a small thing—one top-docs list among many. But it's wildly important because the lists are lying to the public. I know a highly trained Ivy League rheumatologist who only treats what he researches: vasculitis. I treat vasculitis, too—as well or better. The only thing he has over me is the drugs that haven't been approved yet because the institution makes money doing clinical trials. But he doesn't treat rheumatoid arthritis. He doesn't do anything. Similarly, if a patient goes to a tertiary center for a second opinion, that patient sees a student followed by a resident followed by a fellow and then by whomever the attending physician is.

Penn might be the worst place to go to out of the six centers in Philadelphia. The idea that anyone would vote that institution the best and any list would have it at the top is surely a sign of some kind of failure. An accurate list wouldn't put any of the big institutions on top, so the public won't likely see that list anytime soon.

If a self-employed doctor is on one of those lists, it is for one of two reasons: either the doctor is extraordinary or knows influential people. I know this because I am on those lists, I am an extraordinary doctor, and I happen to know influential people. I landed on the US Top Docs list first in 2003 when Muhammad Ali's family called Castle Connolly and said, "This guy saved me and my mother, and he belongs on the list." (I met Ali's family through a mutual friend. Pain was mentioned, and I fixed things rapidly.)

I get onto the lists. A few years later, I did something for the Trump family, and I was told the family members were in agreement with everyone else.

Now the organizations that put out the lists call *me* to ask if anyone in the area should be on the list. I've put about ten people on the list. I have said, "These are excellent doctors, some in my field, some not. They deserve to be on the list because they're fucking good doctors." (I deleted one doctor, and it was appropriate.)

Whenever I send a patient to one of the regional or national top doctors that *I* recommend, the patient always comes back happy. That's opposed to the people who come to me saying they went to nine asthma doctors or this top hospital or that top hospital and they all suck.

In 2009 I was ranked the most influential rheumatologist in the nation. I have no idea how or why, but I know one thing for sure: they got it right. But I am an anomaly. I've been in private practice for thirty years. Many doctors my age retired after twenty-five years or they are getting ready to retire. Right now, the system is so utterly broken that if anyone in medicine over the age of fifty-five is able to retire, they will. They cannot deal with how unethical things have become.

## The Sunshine Act

The hospitals are bad, and the doctors are stymied, but the ethical waters really get murky when it comes to the government, the pharmaceutical industry, and the insurance companies. Take the Sunshine Act, for example.

The Sunshine Act was Ted Kennedy's way of prohibiting the pharmaceutical companies from spending more than a few dollars on lunches with doctors, which was supposed to cut down on a kind of soft corruption ubiquitous in the health-care field. So now instead of taking doctors out to lunch on the pharma company's dime, the companies bring lobster around and make up the names of dozens of doctors! It sounds absurd, but it's true. That said, it's really stupid to disallow the free meals of yesteryear. Only the most unethical provider will use drugs in excess to get a burger with fries!

But that's only a small piece of this corrupt puzzle. Let's say a drug company has—or had—a billion-dollar budget to meet, greet, and feed doctors in order to sell them on the latest and greatest drugs. Now, all of a sudden, such wining and dining is banned. OK, that's good. But where does that money go? Why aren't they putting on educational programs? Why aren't they buying doctors in every field the most up-to-date books and journal subscriptions? Why isn't that money being redirected in a dozen different ways to help doctors help patients?

The money *was* earmarked to feed doctors for decades. So the companies should be awash in extra cash now. Where is the money? Well, the reality is that it's just a slush fund. It's just more money for the executives. In the past, money was spent like water: limos, flights, caviar, Dom Perignon. It was excessive, yet it was industry standard. Now it goes elsewhere, into someone else's pocket. I assure you they are very happy over in pharmaceutical land.

Of course, all sorts of pre–Sunshine Act practices go on unabated; they just take on different forms. When a drug company prepares to launch a new drug, it sets up a task force to look at which doctors to target. After all, these drugs are its products—expensive products—and it has to sell them. If the drug is, for example, an arthritic product, the company blankets all the arthritic-prescribing doctors, and some of the orthopedic doctors as well. After a time, it collect records of every prescription every doctor writes. Then it ranks us. The company record could read, "In New Jersey, Dr. Soloway is the number-one prescriber of drug x and drug y." The next thing I know, I have a drug rep, a district manager, a regional manager, and a regional vice president coming around introducing themselves. They aren't going to take me out to dinner because they can't. That would be unethical and corrupt. But they can sign me up on their speaker's bureau. I used to take part in events put on by the bureau. I would go to hospitals and give lectures, or I'd go to a local restaurant and give a talk. An added level of corruption—restaurants hosting such an event are all owned by the local doctors, who lobby the drug companies to bring their events to their restaurants.

Pfizer and other companies used to wine and dine me to the tune of $250,000 a year to give speeches for them. But as with everything else in the pharmaceutical industry, as soon as the drugs go off patent, the money dries up.

Not every doctor knows about this side of the business (speaking fees are negotiable). The ones who know are the ones who get approached—the doctors with busy practices who prescribe a lot of drugs. The doctors that don't get approached usually have very slow practices and, frankly, they're insignificant.

One bright spot in all of this is that despite the palm-greasing and back-scratching that goes on, I personally don't know of any doctor who has been swayed to prescribe an *inferior* or an incorrect drug, no matter what a drug company has done for that doctor.

Someone might say to me, "Dr. Soloway, why did you write for so much Celebrex? Why didn't you write for Motrin, which was cheaper?" Here is a big inherent flaw in the system and another source of massive waste. Celebrex and Meloxicam, which is Mobic, are the last nonsteroidal anti-inflammatory drugs (NSAIDs) to hit the market. The market is already saturated with NSAIDs. So why were they even allowed to come to the market? The drug companies found one micron of a difference between their drug and the other drugs, and now they're promoting it. I would restrict more than three drugs within the same class, or what are referred to as "me-too" drugs. The money used to develop these drugs, somewhere in the billions, would be better served researching novel approaches to treatments for incurable diseases, whether psychiatric illness or cancers or rare genetic diseases. But having dozens of acetaminophens or ibuprofens under different names is deceitful. And it is stealing from the public.

Now, I do not care how much money is being spent on a paying patient's healthcare. I care that the patient is insured. I care that I'm doing nothing unethical, and that I am treating my patients with the most effective and safe medication. I have reps coming to my office—no lunches, no speaker's fees—saying, "Try this product. It's really good." It takes two years to find out that there is absolutely no difference between this new drug and Motrin. But the FDA approved it; commercials are all over TV for it. Although I'll prescribe the drug, it never should have been developed in the first place—forget FDA approval. Of course it's a fine drug, but it should not have been allowed to be developed. When Motrin, Naprosyn, and aspirin are available, why are companies coming out with this "new" stuff?

The answer is simple, one I will come back to over and over again in this book: money. These drugs are all billion-dollar products, even though there is no significant difference between them and whatever is already available. The drug companies aren't stupid. The marketing is aggressive. Every family doctor has samples in his or her office, and the patients are happy to get them free. Of course, no one gets samples of anything once it's off patent, which is why the speaking engagements then disappear.

When drugs go off patent, the companies drops the price to compete with the generics. But this is how it works. They cash in while they can, and they rake in billions. The CEOs get rich off a drug no one needed, and the system continues to hemorrhage money in waste. Some doctors make some money from speaker's fees or whatever else the drug companies can think to send their way, and everyone goes home happy—except the patient, who gets nothing out of all this, except a drug that already existed. The patient is the last person anyone considers in this system. Another unacceptable problem would be the golden parachutes for exiting CEOs, who in some cases have done little or nothing but drive up prices. Perhaps the golden parachute should be an amount of money distributed over ten years to any and all CEOs, which would ensure CEOs keep their position for ten years and actually do something positive for the company. Pfizer, which I am well acquainted with, watched its stock stay essentially unchanged for over twenty years on the New York Stock Exchange (NYSE), yet many CEOs came and went. Usually they went with $150 million. I value my service infinitely more than the CEO of any pharmaceutical company. I do not know if I have made that much money in my thirty-year career. But if I have, I am certain I earned it.

One overlooked aspect of all this is that medical devices are not regulated in the same way that medical drugs are. Medical-device companies can still wine and dine you and pay you whatever they want because they weren't listed in the Sunshine Act. (Ted Kennedy might have overlooked it. Or maybe he had ownership in a device company! Who knows?)

For reasons I cannot begin to understand let alone explain, one of the injectable drugs that I use, a viscosupplement, is considered a device, as all viscosupplements are. A viscosupplement is reprocessed hyaluronic acid, which is the most common constituent in healthy joint fluid. So when the medical device people come to you, they can try to bribe you as much as they want. They say, "Look, we know that there are seven devices like this on the market. But if you don't think ours is the best, you need to give it a try. Why don't we have you have dinner with somebody who uses it a lot? Maybe we'll go to the White House for dinner and have Dom Perignon and you can get a steak. Hell, you can have a whole cow, if you want!" If it was a pill, that would not be allowed, but for an injectable viscosupplement, bring on the caviar! Unsurprisingly, orthopedics is rife with this kind of thing: steel implantable knees and hips, spinal cord stimulators for pain management, and the list goes on.

In theory these doctors could be getting wined and dined up the wazoo. But for the most part, for a doctor that's really doing well in their practice, this stuff is just a distraction. I haven't met with a drug rep in ten years. I don't want to be on the list. I don't want to accept any food or anything else.

I don't need it. I do not need to hear about the latest and greatest drug or device or technique or practice from the drug companies. There are better, more ethical, and less distracting ways to stay current in the field. I try to go to three courses a year: the Harvard update course and the American College of Rheumatology spring update; I often go to New York University (NYU). Between those three, I hear about the new developments within the field—that have either just been published or will be soon—from the full-time academic doctors.

When biologic drugs first came out, for example, the first one that hit the market was Enbrel, which is a tumor necrosis factor (TNF) inhibitor. About six months later, Remicade came out. But the companies are not allowed to market to you until the drug is actually available. So when Enbrel first came out, I knew of these products from reading about them in the articles rather than from the drug companies and the reps. I was excited to hear about them. From what I was reading, they were going to be game changers in the treatment of arthritis. The studies showed how well they worked over several years of people using them in clinical trials. I started using Enbrel, which was a self-injectable, meaning that I hand the syringe to the patient, who takes it home and injects the drug.

In certain situations, a self-injectable can be convenient. Maybe you have an executive who travels a lot, or a professional athlete. Many productive people don't always have time to sit at my office for an hour. But I noticed the complications of having people inject themselves.

People were injecting through their pants, getting infections, and saying, "Well, my pants were clean; I don't get it." After a few such situations, I knew I needed to find a better way. When Remicade came out, I was very happy because it is administered intravenously, and my patients get it in my office as an infusion. (Say you treat a diabetic who is passed out. If you have the option of mainlining pure sugar through the vein or putting some sugar under the tongue, you take the vein. It works faster and better.)

People will say I'm obviously motivated to do it that way because I'm going to make more money by giving the drugs in my own office. But the patient needs one of the two drugs, and Enbrel is more expensive. So I'm saving the system money and forcing compliance by making sure the process is clean. Plus, I can monitor the patients, and no one will be injecting through pants! I have kept people from needing to be hospitalized!

If you are good enough, you learn about advances in the field the right way. You don't take the word—or the food—of drug reps. You make your own decisions based on your experience. The problem is that not enough doctors are good enough, experienced enough, or knowledgeable enough to know what they don't know. (A Solowayism—The billionaire owns the team, the millionaires play, and the alcoholics watch and get wasted. Yet it's their hard-earned money making the elite wealthier.)

## Consumer Advertising

If plying doctors with food and money to push new drugs isn't bad enough, direct-to-patient advertising dirties the ethical waters even further. This kind of marketing is disastrous. It leads to patients pressuring doctors to use what they see on TV. I have arthritis patients coming to me asking me if they can take a drug for AIDS. "I saw it on TV," they say, "and I heard it was good."

Drug companies have to stop advertising to consumers; instead, they should be educating doctors on what the drugs do. Doctors should read the package insert or talk to a real expert in the field. I'd get rid of the direct-to-patient advertising in a heartbeat. It's like yelling, "Fire!" in the movie theater. When the founders of the country wrote the constitution, they enshrined freedom of speech, but they didn't have to deal with big pharmaceutical companies back then!

I think it's crucial for doctors to be properly educated. The onus is on the doctors to know more than the one trial they read, to really understand what the products do, and to know how to use them in the most correct way possible. Then, doctors might not get the right outcome all the time, but at least they can sleep at night.

Is it unethical to treat a 105-year-old for osteoporosis who comes in asking for a drug the person saw on TV? If you are 105 years old, it's taken for granted that your bones are too thin. You are at risk of breaking them. We also know that bone builders take years to strengthen the bones. Is it worth treating a 105-year-old who has thin bones? Maybe, but only if you think the person is going to live to 125.

Direct marketing to consumers is a terrible idea. It's like teaching physics to a kindergartener. Consumers don't understand what you are talking about. Often the marketing is geared toward somewhat innocuous drugs that people just don't need but that are expensive. It's all in the name of making money for the drug company, and it leads, like so many other things, to waste in the system.

## Reverse Discrimination

A disturbing ethical issue for all US citizens is that American doctors trained abroad are considered garbage, but South Asian doctors trained in their native countries are widely accepted. They don't know our traditions or customs. They are hated by some of their patients. And sadly, they refer within their circle for financial gain. It is reverse discrimination at its finest.

It is not PC or considered ethical for a doctor to discuss income or the business of medicine. If you ask about salaries in your medical school interviews, you will be rejected. It is pitiful, as if you are expected to do all your surgery for charity.

Apparently, you are not to be a doctor to make a solid income? That is odd. Why the hell go to graduate school for $400,000? As an interviewer for medical school, I freely discuss medical economics. All data listed is a lie. Rich doctors are smart and don't share data, while residents make nothing and are included in statistics. Ivy League medical education is only for prospective clinical research where the doctor from only Ivy League or Nepotism University is allowed to get in for $20 million to $50 million in stock options! This is the Wall Street version of medicine, and it dilutes the pool that treats real people. This group is comprised, by and large, of the lazy and unmotivated.

# CHAPTER 2
# BAD GOVERNMENT

## The Definition of Politics

You cannot talk about bad healthcare without splashing around in the squalid swamp of bad politics. As healthcare becomes more and more political—as it's done over the last fifteen years, since the Obama administration, and will continue to do so for years to come—it's important to remember the definition of politics: corruption.

If I'm wrong—and I'm hardly ever wrong—tell me why one has to be wealthy to be a politician. No politician in today's society can give up a job and expect somebody to pay in the hope that he or she *might* win an election. A politician, therefore, has to be a person who can afford to lose money—a lot of money. If someone can afford to lose millions of dollars to get into a political position to make less money than staying outside politics, what does that individual get out of it? The politician gets power.

Today's politicians are not interested in politics for wealth, and they certainly aren't interested in politics for the sake of politics. They are after power, pure and simple. The most skilled politicians acquire and maintain the most power. The least skilled politicians—those who might actually be interested in improving the lives of American citizens—are largely irrelevant. They are neither wealthy nor connected enough to move the needle. This dynamic has colossal implications in every aspect of our lives in this country, not the least of which is healthcare.

Everyone thinks that there are two political parties in the United States: the Republican Party and the Democratic Party, liberals and conservatives, right and left. Right? Wrong!

Let's say I'm suing you and you are suing me. We each have a lawyer, and our lawyers yell at each other in court. They are both trying to win, and neither wants to lose. But an outcome will be reached. In the courtroom, they are bitter opponents. Now let's say I win and you lose. That is, my lawyer outlawyered your lawyer.

Afterward, we see them in a bar having a drink together. We understand now that they were putting on a show in the courtroom—for us, the judge, for society at large. That's the democrats and republicans. They put on a show and then they have coffee together. They are all working toward the same goal, which is the acquisition of more and more power—for themselves and for the system. Congresspersons not on a committee are worthless because they are told who to vote for. But if they are smart, in time, they will dictate who and what to vote for to someone with even less power, and on and on it goes. Further, we don't have a president right now. We have special interests, we have the military-industrial complex, and we have oligarchs.

What we really have here in this country are two political *classes*: billionaires and peasants. The billionaires are split into two groups. If you have $1 billion, congratulations, you are in the first group, the new middle class. If you have more than $50 billion—think Bill Gates, Mark Zuckerberg, Elon Musk—you are an oligarch and, good for you, you are running the country. When Elon Musk decides he wants to buy Twitter, the prediction is Twitter will go from a left-wing tool to a middle-of-the-road tool. But perhaps he has his own agenda to tweet about electric cars and spaceships. Nobody really knows at this point. The federal government is failing us by allowing too much wealth and power. Sadly, we have reached a point of no return where individuals are as wealthy but perhaps not as powerful as the federal government, and those people can no longer be controlled. That may be a good thing, but at what cost? It gives Elon Musk an obscene amount of power. But when you have that much money, you are your own country.

The most powerful politician is nothing compared to the oligarchs. They funnel so much money to force the hands and Nancy Pelosi and Chuck Schumer to get Biden to sign whatever they want; the system is practically set up to do their bidding. Biden can't say no because his family is owned and operated by China or Russia as a result of Hunter Biden's corruption and other illicit relationships. For example, consider the billions dropped off in Iran.

Unfortunately, these people and the politicians they have in their pockets officially make the United States a completely corrupt country from which there is no return to normal. We may have a "democracy" for another hundred years, but it will never operate as a real democracy. It's an oligarchy. Your average person has no power whatsoever.

The other political class is made up of the peasants. I'm a peasant. You are a peasant. We are all peasants. There are three degrees of peasants.

The first class of peasant consists of those able to work but who are on welfare. They beat the system. Good for them. They do nothing and collect checks. They are what I like to call "disposables"—they just don't really count.

The second-class peasant is the "interchangeable." This person has a low-lying government job. One day they're at the VA, the next day they're at TSA, the next day they're at the post office. These people are the walking embodiment of the old Soviet worker's slogan: "We pretend to work, and they pretend to pay us." Our interchangeable peasant may make just a little bit more than welfare and leaves the house to drink beer on the way home instead of *at* the home. It's a life of sorts.

The third-class peasant would be me and you. We work, buy food, eat what we want, and travel to some degree—whether with a bodyguard or alone. But we are peasants nonetheless because we have nowhere near the kind of money that buys any influence these days.

Sad as it may sound, that is the breakdown of our society. There is no other way to look at it. Mark my words: if the lowest man on the totem pole cannot feed his family, there will eventually be a civil war.

How is this class structure related to medicine? We only have to look at who got the monoclonal antibodies first—the upper-level billionaires, the oligarchs, and the president. Chris Christie, Ben Carson, and President

Trump are three that I can think of—not me, not you. It would be months before any of us peasants saw those drugs. It wasn't because they weren't tested yet. (If they were so experimental, they wouldn't be giving them to the president!) It's because they weren't for people like us. We are, to some extent, just as disposable as our welfare group. You can see this across every level of healthcare.

We cannot forget that the oligarchy billionaires have an obvious agenda. Bill Gates owns all the land for food. Jeff Bezos and Elon Musk own the media, the food distribution, and the transportation infrastructure—cars, trucks, and shipping. Mark Zuckerberg owns media distribution. Let's say these three host a fundraiser for Chuck Schumer and demand that their agenda gets signed by the president.

Now that you have a mentally crippled lame duck president, they just pass some papers to him, and he signs.

The oligarch uber-billionaires in America are in many ways just the new Communists. "You *must* do what we say, or you are going to get in trouble." It's not that different from the Chinese model.

People who have that much money don't need more. They scoop up power, and unlike the politicians, who are typically not terribly bright, they're smart enough not to run for office because the office doesn't count for much. It's much smarter for a rich person to give a powerful politician the money.

The heavy donors are giving money to people that are allowed to change, manipulate, and alter the law on behalf of those who are donating. I'm not talking about the $2,500 that many donate. I'm talking about the $25 million or $1 billion—irrelevant amounts of money to people who have $200 billion.

You cannot overlook Obama. The guy's never had a real job in his life. He has no money, but he's got several homes that are worth many millions each. He must be a good investor! I want to hire his stockbroker. The forty acres of oceanfront he acquired in Hawaii during his presidency is evidence enough. There is no other way to look at it.

It's just old-fashioned corruption and it only leads to one place: the New Communism. You eat their food, listen to their media, and there is only one media. For now the oligarchs are teamed up. At some point, maybe the richest will turn on the others.

That's what's nice, in theory, about our constitution. Once you are out, you are out. Of course, the politicians all find loopholes to stick around and stay in power. They hold on to it as dearly as they can. (Say what you will about Trump, but Trump operates like a businessman. He went in and got kicked out. He's not running again. A true citizen politician! Bravo.)

In the meantime, the leftists are pushing a Green New Deal. Do you really believe the United States, with a little over 10 percent of the combined China-India population, is responsible for climate change? This is really nuts. Has the concept of evolution been forgotten? Records for weather have been kept for just over a century, not for one hundred thousand years, and certainly not for one million years. Maybe we are in the variable climate age, like the ice age.

No, the only thing green about a Green New Deal? More Benjamins handed out by government. Where does that lead? Less motivation for work, more government control and overreach. It ends with you and I and everyone else we know being owned by the government. The people have established that they want your leaders only to provide a *perception* of freedom.

If you sit home and you don't work, you get fat and increase your risk of diabetes and heart disease. But you get government insurance. Never mind that government insurance pays doctors less and less or that the good doctors will not take your insurance.

## A Political Awakening

You are probably asking, "Steve, you are a doctor, why do you care so much about politics?" Well, my political awakening came when I opened my medical practice. Before that, I had a sense of how things worked, but in an abstract way.

When I opened my practice, I saw it all very clearly. The light came on when the senator, the congressman, and the assemblyman all came around asking me for a donation. I started asking myself, *Wait a minute, what are these people going to do with my money?* The answer was obvious: "If you pay, we have your back." It's a little mafia: If you don't pay, you get fucked. If you do pay, you may not get fucked. It is protection money. Just look at who gets appointed to ambassadorships—the people that have been paying $300,000 in political donations for years and years. Those jobs are bought and sold like everything else.

I didn't have any background in politics. My family didn't talk about it, and I don't know if they even cared. But I've always leaned Republican. If you are a God-fearing American, the only thing you care about—and the only thing you should care about—is your security, health, and taxes (not in that order).

I got a survey in the mail recently from the Republican Party asking me what I consider to be the three most important issues for the Republicans to pursue. What a stupid question! I said low taxes, less spending, smaller government. Beyond that, a continued alliance with Israel is important. That country protects us more than we do. Israel protects us from ourselves. People don't know that; they don't see it. But it's true.

Sadly, the average voter votes with the last thing they heard on the idiot box and doesn't know what's going on—not even close. The few people who know what's going on are very lucky to have access, and access is power. But you can still have access and not even know what questions to ask. I often don't know the questions to ask. I'm learning as I go. But I do know that if you want to operate a business in a small town, you better know your leaders in that area. You better donate to them even if they're not from your party. One day when the inspector comes, if you can't pick up the phone and call somebody who appointed that inspector, then good luck.

That's how it works.

Doctors are either not paying attention or they don't understand the ramifications of ignoring what's going on politically.

If you ignore what's going on politically, you get what we have now: for the seventeenth year in a row Medicare lowered the reimbursement for an office visit. More and more, nobody wants to participate in Medicare anymore. Maybe a doctor says, "I'll stick with Medicare because I like old people." That's great. But where is the money?

Nobody stops to think how the system is missing so much money. The people on Medicare now, those over sixty-five, are very many—the largest ever on Medicare. How the hell can the system be broke when those people have been paying in this whole time, for decades? Where is the money?

The answer is simple: corruption. (Are you seeing a pattern yet?) Obama and Clinton stole from Medicare, just like they stole from the CIA. The CIA, by the way, with an unlimited budget, does whatever it wants in foreign countries, which is how Bill Clinton robbed the CIA—the money is not accounted for. Most doctors don't even know what the CIA is. They think it's an antibody test.

Medicare is broke, and people still want Medicare for All. Here are a few numbers to consider: We have over 330 million people in the country. About 200 million people are covered in some way by private coverage. Another 100 million are on government insurance. That's 300 million people that have health insurance, and 30 million people that don't. While insurance is limping along and running out of money, it's working for 90 percent of the people in this country. Why would you overhaul the system? Why not just fix the 10 percent?

Over ten million people are covered by two insurances out of these three: government insurance, Medicare, or veteran's insurance. A tremendous overlap is among people who are at least sixty-five years old and the disabled and veterans.

My solution is simple. Take the 10 million veterans off Medicare and go down the list of 20 million uninsured people and give 10 million of them Medicare. At that point you are left with 5 percent of the population who is uninsured, and the real question becomes how to serve the needs of those people. Considering how much waste and abuse there is by the government, they should have to foot the bill and give government insurance to those uninsured.

## The VA

Giving veterans special benefits made sense after World War II and Vietnam, when a cross section of society was drafted. People lost a good chunk of their careers back then, and they didn't volunteer to go. They were called up. Now the military is made up of disposables and interchangeables.

The VA was formed around the time of the Civil War for the soldier who fought with the bayonet and musket. The country needed facilities to take care of injured soldiers from the battlefield. Now the VA has become a guinea-pig farm for humans. Nothing needs approval at the VA. The budget is unlimited. You can learn a lot by experimenting with the veterans.

The soldiers in the days of the bayonet deserved special care because they were fighting for their lives to defend their country. The Vietnam soldiers were drafted. Because they were drafted against their will, the government should have a responsibility to take care of them if they were crippled overseas.

But now we have a volunteer army. If you volunteer to go to the army and you get paid, that's your chosen job. Why are you entitled to more benefits? If we stop getting into these stupid proxy wars, eventually not as many veterans will deserve veteran care. Regardless, I think the VA should disappear now. All the veterans are on Medicare, so they could just go to a doctor. Why does the veteran have to travel fifty miles to go to a VA hospital? When they're already on Medicare, they can go to whoever they want. I'll tell you the reason. Because at the VA hospital, the medicines are free. So when the veterans go to a private doctor, they double dip. They go to the VA for their free medicine, hearing aids, and eyeglasses. It's all free at the VA.

Why do I care? I need medicines for patients, and I see the cost of prescriptions. I say to myself, *The cost could be controlled better if the waste was less.*

All of this is to say that doctors *must* be politically astute. They need to be advised, and they need to be aware. I make a point to put myself in places where I can listen. I hear what people talk about, what issues are being raised in the highest halls of power. I ask questions, not to the point where I harass people, but to fill in the gaps in my knowledge. I read between the lines for the answers when they're not allowed to tell you certain things because they don't want to compromise their power and get in trouble.

Ultimately, it's always a question of waste—and there is a lot of it. The waste is unforgiveable because it's preventable. Getting a VA ID and Medicare ID at the same time gives you two passports to rip off two systems. You are not supposed to have two passports, but the system allows it. Whoever isn't fixing the rule is to blame. I don't blame people for taking advantage of a broken system.

If you have ever wondered why veterans wait years to get an appointment with a specialist, I will explain. In my specialty, we had clinic hours from 9 a.m. to noon. There were six trainees and one attending. We saw six patients per session—forty-two patients per week—in the entire rheumatology section for outpatient appointments. For this reason, follow-ups were scheduled six months or one year later. If patients did not qualify for clinical trials, they may not have been scheduled to follow-up at all. Patients frequently did not see the actual senior physician or the so-called attending physician. That said, if you get a prescription for a free hamburger, the pharmacy will promptly deliver as many hamburgers as you can carry!

No politician wants to touch this topic. But politicians should.

## Medicare for All—Patient Care for None

People discuss universal healthcare and Medicare for All as though they'd actually work. But they will not—they can't. Of course, one reason why universal healthcare can't work is that no one will pay for it. For one thing, it's not in the budget. But trillions of dollars in waste are being spent on other things. Politicians could find the money if they wanted to, but they don't. That's the first problem.

The real reason that universal healthcare can't work is that the good doctors can afford to not accept insurance because the smart people who can afford it will pay the better doctors in cash. Good doctors will not accept patients who have the low-paying shitty government insurance, and bad doctors will, but because they don't know what they are doing they will just make the problems worse. They will, effectively, increase waste in the system and increase pain and suffering in patients, and the cycle will not end. Health-care costs will balloon as the system pumps more and more money into itself to pay for fixing the bad healthcare, all while decreasing the quality of the care.

You'll never have good doctors wasting their time seeing all of these low-paying patients and then getting audited when they see too many of them! You better believe you will have a full-time government auditor there to make sure your notes are good. You'll get a call from the auditor saying, "Oh, you better go look at these three notes. The note doesn't document why you ordered the x-ray. We want to take our money back." No good doctor would put up with it. Only the worst doctors, who have no other choice, would. That's how the system would function—or fail to function.

Doctors are not equal. There are bad, average, good, and stellar doctors. Only a fool thinks otherwise. But the patient always knows. My patients with welfare always say, "My care sucks; no one takes my insurance." There is simply no motivation for physicians to see Medicare patients.

## The RAC Audit

Audits are a nightmare. During the Obama administration, to create money, the government started outsourcing audits to contractors/bounty hunters to go after the doctors that have the highest billing (actually the top 10 percent of builders and needs specialty). In effect, those doctors were told, "We'll take 20 percent of what you collect. You will learn not to be so busy and not to make so much money."

Lucky for me, I had by this time perfected a way of doing 100 injections per hour. This led to an FBI investigation, which I only learned about when former employees of mine were contacted by the FBI. I have a picture of the business cards of the two FBI agents!

The idea behind the audits was to look for doctors who were really committing fraud. But an auditor who doesn't understand what he or she is looking at will think that I, an extremely successful doctor, am committing fraud. I practice the full spectrum of rheumatology. I inject knees and spines—more than orthopedics and pain management, respectively. I am very, very busy. My daughter, doing a clinical rotation at Robert Wood Johnson University Hospital, met a woman that I trained. The first thing she said was, "I love your father. He trained me. He's the best injector in the world."

Some people consider me an artist. My artwork is just crisper than the other doctors'.

Over the course of the last few decades, the trend is such that if a patient has chronic back pain and fails physical therapy and pills, he or she is sent to pain management. Pain management will do an MRI and an epidural. If the epidural works, which it does a small percentage of the time, the patient's pain was from a bulging disk at the level of the epidural. However, I know from experience that 90 percent of the population over fifty-five years old has osteoarthritis of the lumbar facet joints. The symptoms are very typical and classic. I ask the patient two or three questions and know immediately that that's what they have.

I learned how to do injections at the Philadelphia Veterans Hospital by visiting everybody with back pain. When the hospital closed at night, I took the people downstairs and injected medication in them. That's what doctors did at the VA. It made me very proficient, probably the best injector in the world for this.

Pain management does spine injections all day long. It has a very low success rate, not because the injections are wrong but because they are the wrong injections for that diagnosis. If I give you gout medicine every time you have pain, and I am wrong every time, it's either the wrong medicine or the wrong diagnosis. That is the biggest problem that I see. The people that I treat have already had the epidural from pain management. I talk to them and look at their x-ray. I'll get an MRI. I'll do my injections, and they get better. And I save the system money—better success, no ambulatory fee, and the patient is never anesthetized for $1,000.

The best doctors tend to have the most patients. Having the most patients means they have the higher receivables; therefore, they are targeted by auditors.

Audits are triggered from the same diagnosis or level of service used "more often than others," "in theory more than your peers." Since we have Socialist attitudes, both government and private insurance harass physicians, while, remarkably, they tend to not audit large hospital systems.

A wide range of audits exists. For example, meet the Recovery Audit Contractor, or RAC, audit—invented during the Obama years. The RAC auditors (a retired nurse or a janitor—never your peer) will get two or three charts to randomly review by searching for keywords like *severe, chronic,* or *acute.*

If keywords are not seen, the visit is denied. They even deny a flu shot given! You have a visit denied or essentially invalidated. That visit type or level of service is extrapolated over two to seven years, and you get a notification: "You were overpaid by $2 million. Your receivable from that insurance is frozen, and if government insurance was involved, interest of 17 percent, compounded daily, is imposed. You may wish to appeal."

Appeals have five levels. Generally, the bean counter is always right, and you can only be made whole before a judge at the third or fourth or fifth appeal. These audits are criminal-fraud investigations, and most doctors have no idea. If you are very busy, solve problems that everyone misses (common diseases overlooked by the masses are ubiquitous), or are the "doc in the box" (a doctor at a walk-in clinic), you are a suspect!! (Doc in the box and walk-in clinics are notorious for bad care. They see the same patients day in and day out, the patients never get a formal diagnosis, and they never get proper treatment. But as long as the clinic's owners and the government are happy, it won't change. Many patients use such facilities to obtain narcotics and controlled substances.) The process drags on for years and wastes an incredible amount of resources on the part of the auditors, the contractors, the government, and, most of all, the doctors. It has nothing to do with taking care of patients. All of this is really discouraging for young entrepreneurs in medicine.

Other types of audits exist. With the prepayment audit, an insurer will request records before they pay (a great reason for docs to drop an insurance company and patients from their practice). A good doctor these days needs an attorney on the payroll to deal with all of this. I am not kidding.

Recently, a close friend of mine told me he was recently subjected to the prepayment audits for the first time. I told him I was an expert on them, that I'd been getting those for five years. He said, "Well, what do you do?" So I told him: When UnitedHealthcare gives me a prepayment audit, I stop seeing its patients. The company rep calls me to say I have a contract and I have to see its patients. I tell the rep that the contract says I have to get paid. It doesn't say I have to get paid when *the company* decides I have to get paid. It says I have to get paid—the end.

I've given out the home phone numbers and addresses of the decision-makers too. Then I get a call from a lawyer through my lawyer saying, "These people [the decision-makers] think you are crazy. You are insane. What are you doing? You should stop this." I tell them I'll stop it when they leave me alone. It lasts for a year, then the staff changes, and they come after me again. It's deeply unethical and a huge waste of time and resources.

Auditors keep up to 20 percent of the money they steal from doctors. They'll never stop as long as they stand to make so much money. But it's harassment pure and simple. These audits add nothing to the overall quality of healthcare because they go after the good doctors. There are plenty of bad doctors, but the audits will not find them. Audits exist as a scheme to control doctors and take a cut of their money—the mafia model in yet another disguise.

Finally, there are quality audits. The charts are reviewed, and if enough boxes are checked off, the insurance company can receive extra money from the feds! Doctors are actually paid to provide these charts.

There is such a lack of knowledge across medicine these days. For example, because I am so good at what I do, I've established my practice as a back center. All the back pain in my area comes to me. I do more back work than anybody in anesthesia, and nobody in my field is doing back work at all. Immediately, it looks like I am making it up. It looks suspicious. But the most common diagnosis, across the board and worldwide, is back pain.

People played high school sports—they have back pain. People lifted furniture without being careful—back pain. It's wear and tear; it's overuse. There are so many reasons. Everyone who is obese gets mechanical back pain. That and general lack of health are huge contributors. With all the back pain, and because no one is treating it as well as I am or as frequently, my practice invites an audit. I have the skills to help these people, and I am good at it. Why wouldn't I do it?

Some of the rheumatologists thirty miles from here somehow caught wind of the audits—I don't know how people find out—and they were telling patients don't go to me. I am a federal criminal. But I won the audit!

All of that being said, I don't think a lot of outright corruption and fraud exists among doctors. This is why the auditors are targeting people like me, looking for keywords in the charts. Because an uneducated person conducts the audit, the auditor will look at one chart and say, "He didn't document that the pain was severe. And if the pain is not severe, you are not allowed to use Remicade. So we have to deny the visit." They look at one or two more charts. They see what they want, and they don't really understand what they're reading.

The biggest problem with the audits is that they waste an inordinate amount of time. Think about how much it must have cost to investigate me. They lost money on the investigations. Everyone lost money. It's just money wasted.

Fraud and abuse does occur. But an auditor shouldn't have the attitude that everybody who is an outlier is a thief. Maybe the person is an innovative genius (like me!). How about instead of reading the charts, the auditor calls up fifty patients and says, "I want to ask you some direct questions. When you started going to Dr. Soloway, you felt like shit. Two years later, you are on this medicine. Do you feel better than when he started treating you?"

Invariably, they will say, "Much better." What else do you need to know?

I can't bribe my patients to stick up for me. But the system and politics make a mess out of medicine. An entrepreneurial doctor helping patients is made to be the bad guy. Someone must be stealing, goes the logic; it must be the doctor making all this money. Never mind the fact that his patients will all say the same thing: "Dr. Soloway is a genius. He changed my life!"

My success is that I work smart. I found out that if I have a hundred people that need the same thing, I am going to put them in a line, I am going to have them climb on the table, and I am going to do the injection. The minute I am done with the shot, they have to leave. The next one is going to get up on the table. We have people in the room that assist in getting people up and down from the table. If the shot takes me more than two to three minutes, it means I've done something really wrong because that just doesn't make sense.

Pain-management or orthopedic doctors do the same injections that I do, except for some reason they must be done in their surgery center or hospital. That's an automatic $10,000. They automatically anesthetize patients too. That's how they were trained. Why? Maybe they need a rest; I don't know. But when I do them, when I line up a hundred people and do a hundred injections in one or two hours, I don't put anyone to sleep. How's that possible? I don't use anesthesia for the shots because it is unnecessary.

They know they aren't coming for a visit. Once the needle is out, they leave the room. They're coming for a procedure. When they step out the door, the assistant says, "Okay, here is a band aid. You can take it off when you get home. If it hurts, put ice on it. Pain is normal, soreness is normal. If you are not feeling perfect, wait up to five days. If you are feeling 50 percent better, or 30 percent better, or 75 percent better, we want to do it again in three weeks' time." I developed this technique, but because I didn't write an article in the *New England Journal of Medicine*, Medicare will only pay for it once a year now and only after the patient has gone to physical therapy, which, of course, only makes the patient worse.

Many of my patients don't care. They say, "I'll sign the waiver that I have no insurance. How much do you want in cash?" This, I am sorry to say, is the mark of a good doctor in today's overregulated, corrupt healthcare environment.

I might be the only rheumatologist in the United States that does these injections. I will teach my daughter. I see the rewards, both mentally and physically. I am getting compliments from the patients; I'm getting flowers and cards.

Over the past few years the volume of procedures has been diminished greatly because of roadblocks inserted by insurance. These roadblocks include going to and failing that physical therapy. Mind you the patients all complain that physical therapy makes them worse. And while I may get $300 to $500 at most, the same procedure in a hospital may cost closer to $20,000. Why would this nonsense continue? The wealthy simply come and pay cash. But how is this fair to the regular person?

What the insurance representatives try to say when I bring this up is, "Well, you need to get certified as an ambulatory care center." My response is, "Why would I, with the comfort that I have? Why would I waste my time paying an agency to certify me in something I've been doing longer than they've been around?"

"Well that's just the rules—you have to be certified."

That's funny. Before they had rules to certify, I was doing it and making all the patients happy. Yet, the rep would rather they go to a hospital, where it will cost tens of thousands of dollars. There is no explanation for this other than incompetence and greed. It's just so sad.

Doctors don't realize the leverage they have. They are, after all, a group like any other group. All groups are formed out of weak people. Doctors get in groups because they understand themselves to be weak and they feel the need to be with other weak people, so they can seem strong. What do you think a union is? A group of bullies representing the weak.

The government is forcing the hospitals to buy up all the doctors. They put them in a box and guarantee a minimum wage. They can eat, and that's it. The strong doctors are self-employed and creating jobs. But if you are too strong, watch out. You are an enemy of the state, hence the audits, the restrictions, the headaches. The atmosphere is so inhospitable to the strong doctor that many will simply prefer to go work for a hospital or decide against a career in medicine.

It needs to be pointed out because it's true, and nobody else will say it. The repercussions of this will be felt by everyone eventually.

## The Government Grows, You Shrink

One of my favorite Solowayisms is this: As the government grows, you shrink. It's as certain as death and taxes. The more people the government hires to harass self-employed, successful doctors, the more interference, which causes delays due to a lack of hours, of innovation, and of freedom. This is how the VA runs today. If my office were to run like the VA, all of us would be unemployed. The government introduces more regulatory agencies and other hurdles to deal with. If you do not know what I am referring to, try to work for yourself. And if you do work for the government, you are on a fixed income forever, and you certainly have no guarantee of a pension. As any one group acquires more power, the average person has fewer choices, and the doctor has less and less ability to negotiate. Another way to say this would be, "As the government grows, the free market shrinks." You can only see patients during *their* hours of operation, not when you choose to. This is a big disadvantage for anyone needing to see the doctor.

Make no mistake: this government wants it like that, and it will do anything to prop up the system, which requires simultaneously making people more dependent on government for services while running the quality of those services into the ground.

If you are a patient with government insurance, for example, and you go to a clinic, you cannot have the same provider ever. Really, you almost never see a doctor. You only see a nurse practitioner. The patients find it so frustrating. They want me to be their family doctor because I'm the only constant in their healthcare.

The goal of this dehumanizing and degrading system is the following:

- Patients stay home.
- Doctors don't work too hard.
- Insurance CEOs get money.

All of this trickles down:

- Eventually, the patient becomes disabled, either from lack of care or bad care.
- The patient goes on welfare.
- The patient moves into Section 8 housing.
- The patient lives off food stamps.

At the end of this process, which most people are not even aware of, you find that you are owned by the government, and so is your doctor.

On TV, you see the Medicare plan: whatever you need is covered—until you find out that isn't true. The insulin pump that you want? That isn't covered by Medicare. But the government doesn't tell people that some items are restricted.

Medicare is an insurance company, run by the dumbest of the dumb (or the smartest of the smart because they're winning). They are robbing the American people. When Obama came into office, they started a whisper campaign: euthanize old people that cost a lot of money, push them into hospice, push them into the nursing facilities, cut off dialysis for people over seventy-five. These are all very Communist principles. Kill the weak. Lie to the people. With the Medicare Advantage plan, they tell you, "Everything is perfect."

What they don't tell you is if you have Medicare and Aetna or Medicare and Blue Cross, your doctor gets paid Medicare rates, which are the lowest possible. The advantage of Medicare alone is all your procedures are going to be done—not if you have Aetna Medicare because now it's lose-lose for you.

Your doctor gets the least pay, and you get the most restricted rules from Aetna or the other company. That is the advantage? It's more like the Medicare Disadvantage. I would urge no one to have any Medicare Advantage plan, but rather the part B supplement should be Medicaid or AARP.

Of course, the patients that have Medicare and Medicaid don't have a problem getting anything done. The doctor has a problem because if the doctor does a procedure too much, he or she could get subjected to an RAC audit. Remember that the RAC auditor gets 20 percent of what they find on the practitioner even if it's invalid and even if the auditor is off target.

Meanwhile, while I'm working smart and getting punished, the government continues to work stupid and incentivize idiocy. Wherever politics meets medicine, the patient suffers. Before Obama came along—and, believe me, it all started when Obama came along—we didn't have to use computers. Suddenly we had to start using computers. We no longer just pick up the phone and dictate a note.

This was meant to make record-keeping more efficient, right? Wrong again. The computer is there so that doctors can be audited while they are sleeping. That's it. It doesn't help medical care at all.

In fact, there are many hospital systems and offices that are intentionally *not* connected to each other because of the Health Insurance Portability and Accountability Act (HIPAA), the Privacy Act. The right way to do HIPAA is to restrict family members who are not close or people who do not care about the patient. But no two doctors should ever feel uncomfortable discussing the details of a patient. Let's say I have a patient in California and here I am in New Jersey. I call up the doctor in California and say, "Look, I need to know what I need to know." HIPAA blocks that. It's very obstructive and not helpful in any way.

HIPAA is an obstacle that wreaks havoc on the system. You can't get medical records when you need them. But the medical societies are just more far-left organizations working with the government to control doctors. They want institutionalization and cooperation—or else. The lengths they will go to are quite shocking if you know about them. Most people don't.

In the middle of the COVID-19 pandemic, I received $1 million of Medicare money without asking, in two installments of $500,000 each. Out of nowhere in March 2021, my CEO said, "Doc, there is another $500,000 in the checking account. That's a million dollars now. We don't know where it came from."

I said, "Call the attorney. That's why we pay them."

The attorney, our accountant, and lawyer looked into it. They said, "The money is from Medicare; send it back immediately. This is poisonous fruit."

Because of my relationship with the White House, I was able to contact Seema Verma, the head of Medicare at the time. I texted her: "Seema, I just got a million dollars in stimulus money from Medicare, but I never asked for any money. Why did I get this money? What do I do with this money? Provider grant funds are 'no strings attached' yet there are 10 pages of strings that lead to big investigations. And *you* have not provided guidance on how the funds can be used. Please advise immediately. Thanks, Seema!"

Her response: "U can use funds how you want."

I said, "No—the fine print read we 'will be audited.' It's not spelled out anywhere how the money can be used. The rules change daily. I have two law firms and accounting firms advising not to use the money as teams of auditors are being gathered to go after people that use the money 'wrong.' There is no guideline for what is right. What parameters are used? While I don't see many COVID patients, my volume was low because of it. The Medicare auditor will be here the day after we spend it. It feels like a setup. There needs to be a published guideline on where the money is to be spent specifically. Bills, supplies, meds. Obviously, if Medicare publishes that the money can't be spent on ACORN or NRA or abortion, they are crazy or we are crazy. Do you see my concerns and confusion?"

"Use it as you want."

In reality, as I suspected, this was a setup. Had I spent the money on anything other than specific COVID-19 patients, this would have been a felony. I would have been charged and indicted on the False Claims Act and on misuse of government money. It was a sting operation. Anyone who got a tremendous amount of money was set up. Anyone who got $50,000 kept it and put it in their pocket. Nobody used it for stimulation.

It was an easy way to bring me and other successful noninstitutionalized doctors down. Now people in the government would have some concrete evidence to say, "Look, the guy stole a million dollars." Then they tack on every other issue they have, and we negotiate a deal. But nothing really goes away. What they want to stick sticks. I sent the money back.

Doctors were prosecuted for false claims because one of the contingencies of keeping the money was they were supposed to somehow document how it was used for COVID-19 patients. It wasn't like the PPP money, the Paycheck Protection Program, meant to keep a business going.

I must have called twenty or thirty people, friends of mine, colleagues, to ask if they got any money from Medicare. They were people who I knew made $800,000, $1 million, $1.2 million a year. I'm the only one who got anything. Tell me it wasn't a setup! Too bad for them; I'm smarter than they are, and I knew right away something wasn't right. It pays to read between the lines—always know the backstory! (That's another great Solowayism.) The headline never tells the true story.

## Freedom of Speech

One saving grace with regard to politics in this country is freedom of speech. Therefore, I do not have to be politically correct. In fact, it is my right to *not* be politically correct—so long as I don't yell fire in a movie theater. I can be as kind as I want. I can be as sarcastic as I want. I can speak the truth no matter how unpleasant it might be. My political opinions are nothing more than that. People don't need to agree with anything I write or think (though they would be wise to!).

This is a very good thing. Why do you think everyone is trying to come to this country? If this country fails to exist, there will be no free place left in the world.

Perhaps Leftism, Marxism, Socialism, and Communism should be classified in the DSM-5 because it would appear that all the leftists want the freedom to become king. When they do, watch out. Everybody else will have to fall in line.

Unfortunately for them—and lucky for us—the constitution says there are three branches of government. We're safe—for the time being!

# CHAPTER 3
# BAD HOSPITALS AND POORLY TRAINED DOCTORS

## Terrible Training

No one will admit what is increasingly obvious to anyone with a brain: doctors are being trained by unqualified people, and, as a result, their training is poor and their skills subpar. That's putting it kindly. Because of liberal policies and because of a shift in how the elites steal money, we're simply not getting the best of the best these days. (I don't care what liberals think of me. It's completely irrelevant. I want this out there. Someone has to say it.)

During my training, trainees would get fired if we didn't do a rectal exam on any individual in the emergency room. The purpose was to look for blood indicative of colon cancer or an enlarged prostate indicative of prostate cancer. The slogan back then was, "Everybody gets a rectal exam unless there is no finger or no asshole." Patients were checked carefully, and doctors learned more. This is no longer the case. If you have ever been to an emergency room lately, you already know this.

For today's doctor, the exam has been replaced by the computer and the CAT scan. The doctor is forced to spend fifteen minutes (including time on the computer documenting) or less with a patient to make their RVUs. Today's doctor, an employee and not an entrepreneur, works a nine-to-five shift with little interest in seeing patients get better and never develops a long-term relationship with a particular patient. This is a direct result of a shift in training meant to push doctors into hospitals and take away the entrepreneurial spirit that might lead them to think outside the box. In a hospital, you own nothing, and you don't care. You don't even care enough to figure out what you don't know. In private practice, you own everything, and you keep the leftovers, or you are employed, and you have a happy salary that's double or triple what the people at the hospital get for their nine-to-five shift. The same applies to nursing, which is equally dismaying.

It didn't hit home until we became the patients. Doctors who are now getting older become my patients. They're calling me all the time. Their wives are calling me! "Steve, you need to help. You are the only one that understands the system. The new nurses suck, and we're getting tortured! We read *Bad Medicine*! Please!"

The incompetence, depravity, and sheer dishonesty I've seen is absolutely shocking. People don't know how bad it is; they don't know, for example, how deaths are covered up. Somebody can go into the hospital with chest pain, and maybe the person dies by accident. The hospital rep says, "Mrs. Jones, I am so sorry to tell you that Mr. Jones had a heart attack on the table. We did everything possible." It's a lie. The minute the guy's pulse got slow, they threw him in a bag.

But this is the reality. When I was a trainee, I was told I must be a sub-specialist. A generalist would always be overridden by the specialists. A generalist going to court would lose every time. If he or she said something about an EKG, the cardiologist knows more. If the generalist said something about breathing, the lung guy knows more. For joints, the arthritis guy knows more. A generalist was just a triage nurse, really.

Well, now trainers want people to be generalists. Why? To keep them stupid. Today's doctors are told, "You'll come work for the hospital from nine to five." The hospitals get paid more because that's where the doctors are. More docs mean more patients. More patients mean more money. Obama wanted fewer private practitioners and more hospitals, so they started to pay the hospitals more and more, and they started to pay the private practitioner less and less.

Guess what happened? They found out that since the doctors aren't doing more than the nurse practitioner, they could pay doctors *even less*. Now the triage nurse GP has been replaced by the nurse practitioner and the physician assistant. The doctors are putting themselves out of business!

Meanwhile, people believe they have access to care. They do not have access, and access and quality are not synonymous. You go to a clinic, and you never can see the same person twice. You never even see a doctor. You see a nurse practitioner or a physician assistant.

Many patients—more than I could say, or even count—do not want to see a nurse practitioner. They do not want to see a physician assistant. They want to see the doctor—the person with decades of expertise. I will not let any patients see the nurse practitioner until the practitioner is fully established with me first. She will do the stable follow-ups; if there is a problem with it, then patients have to see me the next time. It makes sense.

Now if you go to a family doctor's office or dermatology office, the picture is even worse. You get one dermatologist who owns fifty practices in New Jersey. Each one is staffed with *only* a nurse practitioner who doesn't know anything. The nurse practitioners do the biopsies wrong, biopsy the wrong place, and don't know what to order on the biopsy. They usually just pass out cream. I see this all too often. Patients have a sense of this but often don't understand how bad it is.

## The Field Has Changed

Around thirty-five years ago, an article in the *Annals of Internal Medicine* said if you stop after your internal-medicine residency, which is three years, you can make $80,000 a year. The thinking back then was that a rheumatologist will do two extra years and start off making $10,000 less than the internal-medicine doctor.

Why would anyone go into rheumatology? How are you going to make less doing a subspecialty? The reason that the internists made more was they were taking care of intensive-care patients, administering EKGs, and doing breathing tests. Back then, rheumatologists were just talking to people. Maybe they were gun-shy about needling everything we're supposed to needle.

I was trained by H. Ralph Schumacher Jr., MD (and his team headed by Bruce Hoffman and Larry Leventhal), who literally wrote the book on synovial fluid analysis. For decades he taught synovial fluid analysis at the national meetings. If you were exposed to him, you are prone to stick a needle in anything. I've done it so much that I've perfected my own ways of doing it. It's more efficient, more effective, and less painful to the patient. I get better results. I have patents for several needles!

Thirty years ago, rheumatology was a professional, intellectual field. To make a lot of money, people went into cardiology, where echocardiograms are reimbursed highly. In the gastrointestinal (GI) field endoscopy/colonoscopy procedures generate high revenue and make a lot of money. If they want to make even more money, they did the scopes in their own ambulatory-care center.

A lot has changed. We don't have the really astute, high-IQ people anymore because they're not even going into medicine. They're going into Wall Street if they can. People want to go to Harvard Business School. They don't want to go to medical school. If you get an MBA from Harvard, you'll start off making $100,000 a year at Goldman Sachs, but your bonus could be $10 million.

People say pediatrics is the lowest paid field. That's bullshit because pediatricians live on vaccines. If they give all the vaccines to everyone they can, and they make $200 a visit; trust me, pediatricians are doing fine. The next lowest paid, people say, is rheumatology. I don't know, my tax return might show otherwise because I am paid at the same level as top orthopedics and pain-management doctors. But it's because I was trained properly, I'm self-employed, I haven't been turned into a zombie by a hospital system, and I do everything—absolutely everything—in the field. Plus, I do it better than anyone else.

The American College of Rheumatology description of a rheumatologist states that it's an internal-medicine doctor who takes specialized training in autoimmune diseases—that's it. It doesn't say that not only are they taught about osteoporosis but also they do the testing in the office and give the drug in the office too.

The rheumatologist isn't supposed to be financially motivated, but that's okay for all the other docs. Those rheumatologists financially motivated must be frauds. But am I not allowed to do everything I can to help a patient? Is that financially motivated, even if the patient needs it? Is a doctor not allowed to do gallbladder surgery if the person needs it, because they are going to get paid? They should just let it rupture. Fine, then it becomes an emergency, and it costs even more money.

It's the same thing. I am giving people what they need, keeping them at work, keeping them out of the hospital. One insurance guy—the CEO of the company that has 30 percent of our patients—actually admitted to me that, while the company never did a formal study, he believed that I was saving it money by doing things the way I am. But no one is taught or trained anymore.

My former colleague Audrey put it like this:

If you are anything short of maybe a plastic surgeon or dermatologist that doesn't deal with insurance and takes cash, I don't know how you do it. Unless you have a big contract with certain payers, you can't survive, particularly if you are going to be a primary-care provider; the volume you'd have to see is almost impossible because the reimbursement is not very high. The amount of time you now have to spend in your EMR, I don't know how you would be able to start practice. I would not encourage it either.

I almost feel like: what is the point of going into medicine now, unless you are going to be a plastic surgeon or dermatologist and deal with cash?

A lot of these well-known orthopedic groups don't deal with any insurance at all, and they don't have the overhead of the staff. You pay for everything up front, and you are in charge of getting yourself reimbursed by your insurance company. But a lot of patients, particularly in lower socio-economic areas are not going to do that.

(Continued on next page)

It's very hard to find really good support staff, which Dr. Soloway has. Some of his people have been with him forever. And it makes the flow go better. You set up your schedule for certain things, you try to streamline the process, and you are able to do that volume. Then you almost get punished for doing it. Because the insurance companies are asking, "Why am I paying you so much? How are you doing that many procedures?" When in reality, they should be thanking you for not sending them for surgery when they didn't need it.

He is actually saving the healthcare system.

I worked for a few years as a nurse in New York City in oncology. I went back to get another degree so that I could learn more and do more on my own. I've worked in the hospital setting. I've worked in outpatient. I still work in rheumatology. I see a lot of different things in healthcare. But I'm always surprised and embarrassed about how bad healthcare can be.

One thing about rheumatology, that Dr. Soloway always says, is you have to know enough to be able to recognize what belongs in your field and then be able to refer someone out to where they need to be if it's not a rheumatologic issue. But I can't tell you how many times people come in with things. I was always self-conscious when I first started working like, "Oh, I'm a nurse practitioner, I'm a new grad. I don't know enough." People would come in and I'd think *You've literally been going to doctors for years, and this isn't being addressed, or this wasn't diagnosed, or you need to see this specialist also.* There are definitely a lot of missing links in healthcare, for as smart as some people can be these days, the quality of medicine doesn't match.

It's just different than any other field. Obviously, there are issues in any business. But in healthcare, the work and the training are so grueling for the number of headaches that you get from it. I love seeing patients; I just can't stand the nonsense around seeing the patient.

I could do that all day, every day all day long. It's just the other stuff that takes so much time and kind of ruins it for you.

A lot of the good doctors get pushed out. They switch to the other side—management or pharmaceuticals. But I get it. After a while, your quality of life definitely can be affected. I think that's why a lot of people leave the field, which is a shame because you put so much time and money into your education. Then we have to leave it all behind.

My daughter recently evaluated two patients with pericardial tamponade. They fulfilled all the criteria for this diagnosis. Emergency treatment was required; the patients died. My daughter asked me why the hospital did not do emergency pericardiocentesis. I had no good answer. When I was an internal medicine resident in the 1980s, I explained to her, I did a hundred pericardiocenteses at the bedside in emergency situations either in the ICU or on floors during the night. Here's what she said:

After hearing my father's story and going through the same type of program, nothing is the same today. The emphasis is on saving money—'I am not opening the proper life-saving equipment since recovery of normal health is a bit of a longshot sometimes.' I think it was better in the old days from what he describes. And after reading my father's first book, *Bad Medicine*, I learned a lot about what they used to do, and I see for myself what we are not doing. Working with him on rotation, I was skeptical, but he is not exaggerating. I was a skeptic of his criticisms of the system as well, and the guy (my dad) is not making this stuff up; it's unbelievable.

One of the biggest catastrophes in medicine today is the people who run in and out of the room really fast and speak broken English. They love to take Medicare patients, and they found out how to milk the system by leaving them in the hospital longer and by billing for things they didn't do. There are all kinds of criminal activity, but they're making more than average amounts of money. I have personally witnessed doctors speak with patients via intercom from the main nursing station, never get off the chair, document a note for the thirty or forty people they spoke with, and get paid. Those doctors typically do this behavior after midnight when nobody is really watching. The patients never get to ask questions, and the doctor does not really care what happens.

## The Dreaded Emergency Room

Hospital teaching programs undertrain doctors and they stick them in hospitalist jobs, a nine-to-five shift with a decent little salary. They don't have to worry about the doctors thinking they can do everything because they can't really do anything. Now everything is in place for the hospitals to really start making money.

Patients arrive at the emergency room for healthcare by a well-trained, intelligent professional who should know everything that is wrong—or even potentially wrong—with them. What the patient does not know is who they meet in the emergency room will probably not even be a doctor. It will be a nurse practitioner or a physician assistant, or it could be a medical student or a trainee, such as a medical intern or resident. The same applies to surgery and the other specialties.

So, what have I witnessed? (Let me know if this sounds familiar.) A person comes to the emergency room and is quickly seen by somebody, is triaged, and will either be sent home or admitted. If the person arrives with a medical problem—an asthma attack, shortness of breath, exacerbation of chronic obstructive pulmonary disease (COPD), GI bleed, diabetic coma, thyroid, heart attack, or stroke—he or she will be admitted to the medical service. In the case of a stroke or a heart attack, a neurologist or neurosurgeon is called, and for a heart attack a cardiologist would also be consulted.

Now, this is what goes on behind closed doors. The chairman of the department comes down and tells the resident, "Okay, tonight we are not at full capacity. Fill the rooms. Admit everybody who comes in." Or, "What I want you to do tonight is to fill the hospital to 110 percent capacity." It's no different than what the airlines do. This should tell you that it is all about money. So, all the rooms are filled, including intensive care; telemetry, which is also known as the stepdown unit; and all the emergency room beds, which, depending on the hospital, can be anywhere from ten to fifty. Ten gurneys are lined up in the hall outside the emergency room. Then the hospital goes on what is called "divert." It notifies all the ambulances and all the other agencies that could bring emergency patients not to come, to divert to the next nearest hospital.

Hospital patients are rated by the administration and chairmen. You are worth $500 a day, for example, if you are a patient in the ICU. But you are only worth $100 a day if you are a patient on the general floor. The hospital is looking for ways to make each patient as valuable as possible.

You go to the hospital, you arrive at the emergency room, you speak to the ER personnel, and they ask you who your family doctor is. They then call the medical student or medical resident, and they now have the option of admitting or not admitting you. Let's pretend they decide to admit you. Well, your doctor is out of the picture because the guy admitting you is going to pick his friend or whoever bought him the most booze that month, or bought him the best Christmas present. You can't make this stuff up, but I see it all the time. That's how it works, my friends.

Once you are in the hospital, it's just a question of how much they can milk you for. You get your blood drawn every twelve hours or every day, when, often, that is far in excess of what is necessary. If it is necessary, that patient belongs in the ICU, not on the regular floor. Why do they draw your blood at one o'clock in the morning? Only God knows the answer; I certainly don't. Why does everyone in the hospital have a standing order to have their blood drawn every morning no matter what's wrong with them? Again, I'll defer to God on this one.

But that's only the beginning of the story. So much money is thrown out in the system, at every opportunity. Let's say a person has facial plastic surgery and that if it is done in a private office it costs $50,000. The reality is, if a person gets facial plastic surgery for $50,000, they pay the surgeon the $50,000 and the surgeon pays the anesthesia person $5,000. He pays his nurse $2,000. If he does one or two of those a day, he's rich.

Now let's switch, and say, "I'm not going to get a facial plastic surgeon with a private office; I'm going to go to the hospital and get heart surgery." The procedure is the same $50,000, except now you've got the hospital fee, which is $250,000. The anesthesia fee is now $25,000. Instead of the three full-time nurses who really know what they are doing, you've got seventy-five nurses who have no clue what's going on. They walk in and out of the room all day. They say, "I'm sorry, can you tell me what's wrong?" If you don't answer, they walk out. They order blood nonstop. They're giving people saline rather than heparin flushes, causing people to get unnecessary deep vein thrombosis, which leads to complications and longer hospital stays. They are leaving in catheters, IVs, and everything else too long. It's a mess of incompetence, and there is a total lack of accountability. But the hospital gets paid, so everyone is happy.

The bottom line is that hospitals are paid extra compared to a private doctor with the lower-paying insurance, such as Medicaid. While most doctors will not accept this due to low reimbursement, the hospitals get the Medicare rate, which is two or three times the Medicaid rate. This limits patients' choices regardless of what the latest politicians are selling.

Another strategy hospitals use is admission and discharge. Remember way back when a person would be admitted for a bad problem, perhaps a heart attack, and stay a week or so in the hospital? These days, people are tossed rapidly. If admitted for observation, you are kicked out just short of twenty-four hours. Why? Too many short-term admits or readmissions may result in less money for the hospital.

Here is a situation you should find disturbing. I witnessed a physician who had no practice; he simply saw patients at the hospital. However, this has nothing to do with a hospitalist. This is just a physician who would go to the emergency room and take emergency-room call. Anybody admitted without a primary care physician gets assigned the doctor on emergency-room call. So, an ICU admission gets that physician $500, and a discharge from the ICU gets the physician another $500, and every day that doctor says hello to the patient results in $350, while other people manage the case.

I have watched somebody become uberwealthy—by doctor standards—just by milking the system in this way. He admitted everybody and kept them in as long as possible. Nowadays, it is a little more troublesome because the insurance companies will not pay for the unnecessary time in the hospital, but, believe me, it still goes on. Have you ever heard of a *courtesy consult*? Well, if you are a patient at a teaching hospital, your teaching team is going to be your admitting doctors and your family doctor, who doesn't generally go to the hospital. If he happens to come by, he says to the teaching team, "That's my patient; I want a courtesy consult." So, he collects $250 and writes a note on the chart. Now, I'm not sure if that's stealing or stupidity, but it falls under each category as far as I'm concerned.

## Getting a Proper Diagnosis

Even the specialist training is bad. Everyone is told they're crazy because the doctor doesn't know what's wrong with them. Many of my patients have been to a minimum of three specialists in the same field over the course of five years. They come to me one time and get a proper diagnosis.

I'll give an example: A patient comes to me and tells me that they have fibromyalgia. I talk to them, ask them this, that, and the other thing, and I conclude the patient doesn't have fibromyalgia. The patient looks at me perplexed. I say, "You should be ecstatic. You thought you had fibromyalgia for five years. You went to three rheumatologists, all of whom confirmed it. But you are still just as lousy as you were five years ago. Now I'm telling you that you never had fibromyalgia. This is what you have. Come back in a month or two. I think you'll be better."

I truly believe that your lawyer, your accountant, and your rheumatologist are the three most important people in anyone's life—assuming your rheumatologist is even half as good as I am! I could tell stories all day long for a week about the terrible treatment patients have received before they found me.

Take a psoriasis patient I saw not too long ago. The patient had erosive joint disease, left first metatarsophalangeal joint (MTP—the big toe), and saw an MD and had amputation; cultures were negative. The amputation was unnecessary. Infectious arthritis, crystals such as gout, and destructive arthritis, such as rheumatoid or psoriatic arthritis, may all look the same. If an orthopedist rather than a rheumatologist is called, fluid may not be aspirated, crystals will be overlooked, and the patient will have unnecessary surgery.

Or consider an inflammatory arthritis patient who was referred to me for rheumatoid evaluation. Orthopedic surgeons said the person needed emergency carpal tunnel surgery bilateral, which unfortunately occurred. The orthopedic surgeons were smart. They knew I would cancel the surgery and treat the patient. I suggested treatment of psoriatic arthritis and nail changes with biologic therapy, TNF inhibitor with methotrexate. The patient refused, citing that Otezla looked better on TV and had no side effects, while the methotrexate package insert looked dangerous.

Then there was a patient with palpable purpura seen in the hospital. The patient needed a punch biopsy with immunofluorescence. Instead, I was told by the dermatologist that they do shave biopsies. (She does not know her nickname is "the Butcher.") She left two horrific scars. I did two biopsies, one for immunofluorescence, one for hematoxylin and eosin (H&E). They never did immunohistochemistry. The proper way would be to have a small punch biopsy, two to four mm, and all three tests are done on that biopsy alone. This is strictly for palpable purpura, as there are lesions that should be biopsied in the center and the edge of larger lesions.

Another patient came in with a rash on both hands, which she had for multiple years. Years ago, she went to a dermatologist, who opened the computer, showed her a picture of a similar rash, told her that is what she had, and basically said she should deal with it. She then tried to biopsy the rash, but instead of doing a punch biopsy she cut off some skin with scissors. The dermatologist called the patient later because the biopsy was insufficient; she had to return for a second visit and a second biopsy, for which she was charged. At no point was immunofluorescence or immunohistochemistry done, and the patient was discharged from the dermatology practice.

The patient came to me five years later on a referral from her GP, who felt that the rash could be autoimmune and that the rheumatologist should be involved in the care of the patient. I witnessed an annular rash on both hands. The left hand had a new lesion; the right hand had several spreading or migrating lesions that were injected by the dermatologist years ago and had scarring and blanching of the skin but no improvement of the rash. I attest this is 100 percent accurate—and 100 percent horrifying!

I received a call not long ago from a colleague regarding a thirty-four-year-old white female who "looks like she's dying." She couldn't stand up, couldn't talk, was stuttering, couldn't feel the right side of her face, had lost vision in her right eye, had no strength in her legs, and had burning in her upper abdomen, chest, and back.

With that information alone, I diagnosed transverse myelitis and asked her to come to my office the next day, which she did. I was able to confirm my diagnosis in person. I later found out the patient had demyelinating brain lesion that she was told was from possibly migraine headaches or something else benign. She underwent plasmapheresis in the past for an unknown reason.

The symptoms I described had never occurred until recently, and they were progressively getting worse. She will have a differential diagnosis of lupus, vasculitis, neuromyelitis optica (NMO), and MS. She will need a lumbar puncture; cervical, thoracic, and brain MRI with contrast; and pulse steroids and cytoxan, all as soon as possible. This is negligence and a terrible dereliction of duty by any and all doctors who have seen her in the past.

Here, in her own words, is the infuriating and all too common story of another patient, KB:

In March of 2020, right when the pandemic hit, I noticed that I just wasn't feeling normal anymore. I didn't know what to do. I went to my primary-care doctor, and I told them I had just pain in all my joints. They told me that they thought it was just stress due to the pandemic; they said to just wait a few weeks, and I'd be okay.

I just kept getting worse and worse. I was only thirty at the time and very active. I worked out all the time. The older people in my family said I needed to see a rheumatologist. So I went to a rheumatologist in Georgia, where I live, and I told her that I just hurt everywhere. But I didn't have any inflammation. Now, I have a lot of tattoos, and it's hot in the south, so I'm wearing short shorts a lot. I could tell the doctor took one look at me and thought I was lying. She was so dismissive. She looked right at me and said, "There is nothing wrong with you, and you need to leave."

So I went to my car and just googled who were the best rheumatologists. Dr. Soloway's YouTube popped up. I sent him a message, and he messaged me right back. He said, "Go back and tell them you need a blood panel." I went back in and told her. They ran a blood panel, and it came back crazy bad. I was really, really sick with rheumatoid arthritis. When she called me on the phone with the results, I said, "You were so dismissive of me when I told you I was sick." And she said, "I've met you?" She had no clue.

She put me on methotrexate and told me to start with that. But I didn't even know what rheumatoid arthritis was, and no one bothered to explain it. I thought the medicine was like an antibiotic. I would start taking it, and two days later, I would be cured. Nobody told me I had to be on it for twelve weeks before it was in my system. No one told me this was about to be a lifelong journey at all. I thought it was like strep throat. I thought I was going to be okay.

After about a week on the first drug, I called the doctor back and said, "I'm not getting better. I'm not taking this anymore." They sent me to a new doctor, who changed my medicine. He never told me it would take weeks to work and just trust the process. Nobody ever said that.

Over the next few months, I started the whole journey into this illness. Being so young, it's not like any of my friends have anything like this going on. I learned everything about my disease through Dr. Soloway's YouTube videos. Anytime I had a question, he would always answer me right back. Finally, in the summer of 2020, I was really sick. I asked him if I could come, if he would just evaluate me. He saw me that week. I flew up and met him. I've been going to him ever since.

But when I met Dr. Soloway, he did a lot of bloodwork, and he found out that he thinks it's psoriatic arthritis. He explained everything, and he put me back on track. I remember very well when Dr. Soloway asked what infusion I used. I said, "Inflectra," and he said, "I don't even give that. That's (biosimilars) akin to generic." He changed all my medicines, but I still have to have infusions, and being in Georgia, those infusions have to come through my insurance company. It wasn't like he could just send me home with an infusion and a needle.

I rocked along for a couple of years, just with his care. Then in January of this year, I got just sicker and sicker and worse than I was whenever I first got sick. I had no clue what was going on. I went to my rheumatologist here in Georgia because that was the cheaper insurance thing to do. My blood tests all came back that I had drug-induced lupus from the infusion my rheumatologist was giving me in Georgia. I called Dr. Soloway and asked what to do. And he said, "You need to tell them they've got to stop that infusion because it's making you sick. Ask them to change it to something else." They said no way. They said it was too expensive to change to something else. And that was it.

It all goes back to the insurance company. I'm at their mercy when it comes to the infusions. Dr. Soloway told me I need Enbrel. When I went back to my rheumatologist here in Georgia, and I said I need Enbrel, he said, "There is no way you are ever going to get that. They're never going

*(Continued on next page)*

to approve it." So I asked the pharmacist, "Do you ever see Enbrel get approved?" She said, "You could never afford it."

Dr. Soloway actually gave me an Enbrel while I was in his office. I was 1,000 percent better five days later.

I've flown up to New Jersey six times in two years to see Dr. Soloway. I'm totally better now.

Sometimes I think about what I would have done if I had never met him. I would have just thought that this was my life. Every time I went to my rheumatologist in Georgia and said, "I'm not getting better," they said, "Neither is anyone else." And they would always tell me I could get a referral to the pain clinic. They had no problem giving me a referral to the pain clinic. Dr. Soloway said, "Do not do that."

The more insane part is I have a thirteen-year-old who in 2020 also got crazy sick. She has Asperger syndrome, but she's your normal run-of-the-mill kid. I took her to the pediatrician and said she can't move her hands. She had obvious inflammation. They sent us to the Children's Healthcare of Atlanta, and we met with their rheumatology team. Obviously, I went through my whole story, and they told me that it was an oversensitivity to pain due to her autism. And there was absolutely nothing wrong with her. They said, "Maybe she's doing it for attention because she hears what you are saying." I said, "She can't get in and out of the bathtub by herself. What teenager wants their mom's help doing things like that?" They never believed me or her.

And they said, "We can send her to counseling, and we can send her to pain management, but your journey has nothing to do with her journey." The first time I met Dr. Soloway, before the end of our appointment, I said, "Can I bring my daughter to see you? He said, "What's wrong with your kid?" I said I didn't know, but something is wrong. She's not lying.

He saw her, and he was the first doctor who really listened to her. He put her on medicine in January and she's a completely different kid now. She can swim. She makes all kinds of tiny bracelets and jewelry. That sounds small, but she used to not be able to hold a toothbrush.

> I remember the first time Dr. Soloway explained everything and told me about the treatment, I asked how long I'd be on it. "Forever," he said. I just died. But he was so nice. He said, "You are with a really good team. It's going to be fine." And he's right. It'll be fine.

## Bad Training = Bad Medicine

My daughter, mentioned above, is a third-year medical resident at a community hospital. It is my opinion that the government is paying hospitals to interfere with medical education and keep the doctors inexperienced and stupid, which will lead to a forced socialized system. The residents at the hospital where my daughter is a third-year medical resident recently had dinner with a senior official from the hospital who indicated that they should not go into private practice but rather should work for the hospital. My daughter has had minimal exposure to sick patients in the intensive-care unit because there is an intensive-care-unit team, little exposure to doing procedures such as central lines because there is an IV team, and very limited exposure to critical-care medicine and emergency medicine due to the so-called teams that have been assigned to dilute the knowledge of an internal-medicine specialist.

When I was a resident, nothing was off the table, and students learned and did everything. The graduating classes of the past ten years are not prepared; students are sabotaged in their education. This can only be due to the financial incentives from the government to the hospital. The government gives hospitals money. The money is for doctors and the hospital to share. This is why teaching hospitals just appear!

The medical care most people receive is obviously appalling. So why do so many patients put up with it without questioning?

The answer seems simple. Training is now terrible. Nurses and medical trainees are only required to document notes. They do not see the patients; they do not know the patients. They do not have any clinical judgment. They frankly have no idea what they're doing and, in many cases, don't belong caring for patients at all in any manner. As extreme as this sounds, this is the truth, and if you don't believe me, it just means you have never been a patient before. Being twenty-five years old and healthy is a dream! I promise you, it will not last. At fifty, your engine light may come on!

Why is everybody brainwashed? Why is every urgent-care, emergency-room, and family physician referring all joint pain to orthopedics when 98 percent of all joint pain is nonsurgical? In my area, they have no excuse not to be acquainted with me. I've been practicing for three decades. I've treated tens of thousands of patients with astonishing success.

Why is it that spine surgeons train as neurosurgeons yet orthopedics schedule that work as well? Is there a financial incentive? Or is it that, as I once found out, getting occupational-medicine contracts requires bribing individuals working at these companies? Yes, you read that correctly. Your company picks the doctor who is the "highest bidder" to the insurance company that covers the injuries at your place of work. You think you have a choice, but the choice has been made for you. You don't get a choice at all. Why are inexperienced doctors perpetrating delusional lies upon patients who don't know any better?

In the 1980s we were all encouraged to be subspecialists, somebody who knew more than anybody in the given field. We were trained—the best of us—to want to be the best, to know everything there was to know, to treat patients to the absolute limits of abilities, which were considerable. Now doctors are pushed to extending their residency into a career of nine-to-five residency, effectively eliminating the self-motivated thinking man or woman in favor of the relative-value-unit-driven, dumbed-down robot doc. The result is bad medicine.

# CHAPTER 4
# BAD PHARMA

## The Drug Patent

Dr. Oz called me not long ago. He had read some of my book and thought it was really well done. He asked, "If I win the Senate, what do I do my first day in office to help healthcare?"

"Slow down a little there," I said. "That's not something I can answer impulsively." I thought about it for a second and said, "We need to extend drug patents from twenty years to forty years, so that the prices can be lower. The drug companies will still be able to make their money back, but the drugs would be more affordable. We'd have to prohibit companies from making a fourth, fifth, sixth version of the same drug. It's stupid to have ten companies making Tylenol. Billions and billions of dollars are being thrown out. It's money that would be better spent on researching novel therapies—as long as that money can be made back."

Once a product goes to the FDA—if everything goes properly—approval is granted, the drug manufacturer is allowed to start distributing a drug, and the manufacturer is issued a twenty-year patent. From there, it generally takes six to seven years from the patent date to bring a drug to market. The manufacturer automatically loses that much time to make the money back. Once the drug starts to sell, the company has thirteen years to gouge the prices and make as much money as possible. It can usually gouge the price really good for about ten years before two or more other companies make a competing product. Those companies, of course, are in the same situation, so they need to keep their prices really high. At the twenty-year mark, the patent runs out, and companies can begin to make generic versions, which compete with the original drug. The original drug no longer makes money, and in some cases the companies stop producing it, which is ridiculous because over the last fifteen years, people have come to rely on it.

Now, if a patent were to last for forty years, the drug companies no longer have to gouge the price to make their money back. Instead, they can set a fair price and make their money back over a longer period before the competition can begin to eat away at the same market.

This would be great for patients. The only people it would affect negatively are the drug company CEOs, and they would fight it tooth and nail. I have noticed more and more of them retiring after eighteen months and leaving with $150 million. A good leader used to stick around for ten, fifteen, or even twenty years. A good CEO has really made something and deserves the big package. But someone who comes in and retires a year later? He or she doesn't deserve it but has figured out a way to exploit the system.

For the first ten years after Remicade came out, I was paying, let's say, $1,000 per vial and being reimbursed by the insurance companies at $1,050 per vial. Once the patent ran out, biosimilars came along, and now I buy the same Remicade for $365 and get reimbursed $400.

So let's just pretend that manufacturer knew it had a forty-year lock on this drug, and it started the price at around $600. It can make its money back over a longer period, but the price never goes too high, and the insurance companies don't go crazy. At the same time, I'm getting paid based on the time it takes for the infusion and whatever the profit on the drug is.

But no one wants doctors to be pharmacists. (Some barely want doctors to be doctors, but they certainly don't want them to be pharmacists.) In fact, if I want to dispense drugs in my office, I have to hire a pharmacist, which is pure politics. Doctors should know more about the drugs than pharmacists. In the old days, a pharmacist would count the pills and give them out. It was safe, presuming the person counted the right pills. Now a pharmacist is required to get a PharmD just because there are so many pharmacists—so becoming one has been made harder, but there are still too many. So now, instead of pushing pills, they work in hospitals, supposedly advising on drug interactions. If you are a halfway normal doctor, you should be the one telling the pharmacist about interactions, not the other way around.

This is all in an effort to control healthcare by overregulating it to death—a divide-and-conquer strategy. Don't let any single health-care professional get too smart, too useful, or too entrepreneurial. Keep all doctors in their box or corner; keep them busy and distracted, and they are easy to control. Once you see it, you can't unsee it. It's ubiquitous and dangerous.

Speaking of the political-pharmaceutical-insurance complex, the other thing Dr. Oz spoke to me about was how slow the process is for the government to study and approve drugs. It takes years, and only one in twenty drugs ever get to market. I told him the truth: "If the government is involved, it will never be as good as if private entities are involved."

With the government, a limited number of people work on these things, and there are *always* political games. The people in the FDA who are voting on approval are friends with people in the pharmaceutical industry, and they are being twisted and bribed in every direction. People fudge articles, make data look a certain way, so they can get drugs approved by the FDA. People fudge data so that they can skew populations of doctors to use a protocol that will favor an algorithm that will lead back to their medical device.

Government people do not make a lot of money but think they are very powerful. So how do they exploit the situation for their own financial benefit? They turn it into a bribery ring.

I'll give you a true example of how twisted the pharmaceutical industry is. When Janssen Pharmaceuticals launched Remicade, it was in a rush to get it out because Enbrel came out first, with a six-month head start. Enbrel is self-injectable; Remicade is IV only. Humira was third on the market. (Humira is the most prescribed, due to deals and ads.)

But within five years, Humira had the lion's share of the market. Why? Pharmacy executives said, "We have to get this drug out there. So we're going to start discounting all of our cancer products to the facilities that buy them, and we're going to take a little hit on the cancer drugs with which we're cleaning up. Now we're going to look like good guys, and we'll make Humira a $12 billion drug." That is exactly what happened.

Now commercials are on the idiot box every ten minutes saying, "Humira is the 'number one prescribed drug.'" Well, that's fine. It's not the *number one* drug. It's just the number one *prescribed* drug—big difference.

It's not the best drug. It's most certainly not the least expensive drug. (Those pharma guys aren't stupid!)

People think drugs that can be given at home—the self-injectables—and drugs that can only be given intravenously in an office or hospital setting are both needed. So the self-injectable must be the cheaper and the IV must be the more expensive. Lo and behold, if you go to the medical office, which is a comfortable setting for receiving intravenous drugs and leads to better compliance and therefore better outcomes, you'll find out that the higher dosing of Remicade, given intravenously at the office setting, is cheaper than any self-injectable drug. You might think that's odd, but it isn't. The pharma people know doctors are not investing in places to infuse, which I did. They know that hospitals are not storing or stockpiling the drugs because there is not enough need to lay out money. So they're not getting a good deal on purchase, and they're not getting a good rebate.

The self-injectables are pushed hard. But in my experience, in the office there is complete compliance with no infections, and patients stay out of the hospital, which saves the system a lot of money. You are also helping people improve their quality of life. I've seen it throughout my entire career.

Now, Aria is the patent extender of Remicade, essentially. It was FDA approved in a less-than-optimal dose because the medical director at the time wanted to hurry and push the drug out.

It's double the price of Remicade. Unsurprisingly, all the insurance companies have taken Remicade off as their tier-one drug, and they insist on using what's called a biosimilar. For our purposes, biosimilars are generics.

Let's talk about biosimilars. These drugs are protein molecules that are too large to make into a pill, so they are parenteral instead. If you were to drink the IV, which you can with some medicines, the hydrochloric acid in the stomach would destroy the product. They must be given parenterally.

By definition, biosimilars are not the same as the original drug. They're *similar*. Regardless, the insurance people will say, "You have to switch your patients from Remicade" to whichever biosimilar they have on their formulary. They'll write me a nasty letter saying that next month, I'm not allowed to use Remicade anymore. I have to use the biosimilar. But I'm smarter than that. I look on their first-tier list and I see a more expensive, branded, patent-protected drug. They told me to switch all the patients, so I do. Except instead of switching to a biosimilar, I switch them to a reference drug, which is twice the price, and I double my income.

"Wait, you can't do that," they say.

"Yes, I can. You know why? Because I documented that the insurance company forced me to change. The patient refuses to go on a generic drug. I switched them to your first-tier drug."

In addition to that, the company that makes Remicade cut the price to compete with the generics, low enough to match the biosimilar or generic price. This is a crucial part of this story—and the story of many drugs. There is no difference in price between any of the biosimilars and their reference drugs, *and* there are more than three reference drugs, which represents an enormous waste of money.

Nobody should have to use a lookalike drug if already on the one that works. Cost is no longer an issue. Remicade is the cheapest drug—if infused at the office. But no one can seem to put two and two together. Sadly, due to a phenomenon called immunogenicity, a patient may not respond to the drug after having success and then stopping, hence restarting may be an effort in futility.

Here's another example: I've been taking Nexium for five years, since my bout with cancer. My tumor was producing gastric acid, which led to acid reflux. I am therefore committed to a lifetime of proton pump inhibitors. AstraZeneca, which makes the Nexium, used to make a bottle of 1,000 for $7,000. When AstraZeneca's product went off patent, it no longer made a bottle of 1,000 because nobody would buy it. People would buy the generic.

As a patient *and* a doctor, I will not say the generic is inferior. I will say that the generic is different. Is it ethical to change a person from a reference drug to a generic when he or she has been on the reference drug for ten years, just because the drug is off patent?

If the company makes it, you have to pay out of your own pocket because the insurance company says, "We're not paying for that. You are going to get the generic." Three and a half years ago, I bought that bottle of Nexium from my wholesaler for the aforementioned price. Recently, when that ran out and the bottle of one thousand was no longer produced, I did the next best thing: I bought ten bottles of ninety pills, and the price for the 900 pills was over $8,500. But I got another three-year supply and nobody knows I'm on it. Frankly, I'd rather pay more. But if I went to the pharmacy with the prescription, I'd hear "Sorry, it's only generic." Talk about terrible healthcare. It happens all the time, and people don't realize it.

## Generics

But none of the aforementioned compares to the depths Horizon Blue Cross sunk to when it sent a letter to all their patients offering a $50 gift card to some place like Dunkin' Donuts in exchange for having their medication switched from the proper drug to the generic drug:

> Great news! You are eligible for a one-time $50 gift card if you switch from a brand-name medicine to its generic equivalent. . . .
>
> Switching to a generic is safe and easy. When you choose a generic prescription medicine, you can expect the same safety and effectiveness as the brand-name medicine, but generally at a lower cost to you. You are also eligible for a one-time $50 gift card for each brand-name drug listed below that you switch to the generic equivalent. . . .
>
> Your current medicine: Xanax XR TAB 1MG
>
> Generic equivalent: Alprazolam TAB ER 24HR 1MG

The whole concept is just completely unethical and immoral. To make a switch that will supposedly save the company tens of thousands of dollars, you would think it could offer more than $50. In fact, if it offered everybody free insurance or $5,000, it would still save a ton of money based on some of the drugs available.

This, however, does not mesh well with the nine-figure departure package obtained by the CEO of each company. Once three drugs are in any one class, no more should be allowed; companies should be forced to spend money on novel treatments and attack afflictions that have no treatment at all at this point. Anything else is robbery, pure and simple.

# CHAPTER 5
# BAD INSURANCE

So far, you know politicians are bad, doctors are bad, hospitals are bad, and the pharma companies are bad. I know what you are thinking: *the health-care industry is a joke.* But I haven't even gotten to the worst part yet—the insurance companies! The insurance companies harass everyone—doctors, nurses, patients—incessantly. They are without question the biggest problem in healthcare right now. They force me into fights, which wastes enormous amounts of time that would be far better spent treating patients.

We have more than thirty chairs in my office. We have six full-time nurses, and right now we're being harassed by AmeriHealth, which is owned by Independence Blue Cross.

Here is how the story started. In the mid-1990s I explained to the CEO of AmeriHealth New Jersey at the time, Judy, that in a rural neighborhood people can't go up and down flights of stairs to get X-rays and bloodwork. I told her I do X-rays, blood, shots, everything here in the same office. It's too much running around and people won't get the testing completed. She liked my idea of doing it all in one place.

I said, "Well, this is how rheumatology is practiced." She said it wasn't what she was used to. At that time, rheumatologists with that insurance company couldn't even do their own X-rays. That's an orthopedic thing, according to insurance companies. But orthopedics looks for fractures, and I look for everything else—not for fractures. The radiologist doesn't know the patient, and unless you have a relationship, as I do with the local bone radiologist, that person doesn't even know what to look for.

For example, an MRI is ordered by an orthopedic surgeon or a neurosurgeon, and the report comes back, noting a herniated disc at a certain level. Now, the patient could have profound arthritis—this would be called facet arthritis—but it's not mentioned. But you can't *not* mention the arthritis just because you don't think it's important. The neurosurgeon is looking for a disc or a nerve to decompress. I'm looking for everything, including arthritis that I can perhaps inject or for which I can ease the pain.

The bone radiologists that I work with are very in tune with what I am looking for. In fact, the chief of radiology, also a bone radiologist, at the local hospital where I'm the chief of rheumatology was one of my teachers thirty-five years ago in the Philadelphia VA. That's a good situation.

In any case, Judy left AmeriHealth, and I developed a very good relationship with her successor, Frank, who is not the CEO. He is the senior medical director. Unbeknownst to me, he answered to someone in Pennsylvania, not New Jersey. (Who owns these companies doesn't affect me—until there is a problem, and then it's very important. It's good to know what's further on up the chain.)

At one point, I said to Frank, "You need to come out and see our office. We do X-rays, blood draws, and infusions. We are state of the art, and we're cheaper than every other place, no matter where."

Many people don't realize that when you go to the hospital or an ambulatory care center, you are often getting two copays. There is a copay for the doctor and one for the facility. When you go to my office, there is just one copay because it's just an office. So it doesn't matter what we do to you at the office. It's part of our field, and that's what we do. Now, a large majority of rheumatologists do not infuse in their offices or do their own X-rays. Very few have ever read their own X-rays.

And because I am capable of doing all this stuff at the highest level, there is a witch hunt against me! I just passed my rheumatology boards for the fourth time. I'm fifty-nine years old. This is my thirtieth year in practice. I'm the chairman of rheumatology for three hospitals. Arguably, I believe I'm the best clinical rheumatologist in the world. But I don't have a resume of five hundred pages because I'm not a clinical researcher, and my success makes people insane. It's unbelievable, actually.

Frank at AmeriHealth and I got along very well for a few years. He came out and loved the facility—*loved* it. I said, "Frank, I want you to put me on the list of the preferred places that your insurance wants people to go to because it's the cheapest."

"I like the idea. I'll go back to my superiors."

"I thought you were the superior."

He explained about the people in Pennsylvania and so on. But I was made to believe that after COVID was over, the higherups would come out and approve me to be one of their preferred sites.

The exact opposite happened. Instead, I got a letter from this guy's boss, a doctor who is probably too incompetent to practice, which is why he's working at one of these places. He's not an older guy; he's just a guy who made a career of making doctors' lives shitty—to empower the institution, if you will. The letter said, in so many words, "Hey, you are doing X-rays, and you are not even allowed to do them. What's your certification?"

I got on the phone and said to someone there, "I've been doing X-rays with AmeriHealth patients for twenty-eight years out of my thirty-year career." I negotiated that with Judy. I had demonstrated to her that I'm perfectly capable of doing X-rays. Here it is, years later, and nothing's gone wrong. There has never been an adverse outcome, a death, or a misread or missed cancer, and people are happy with the treatment.

"But you are a rheumatologist; you are not allowed to do that."

"You can't talk to me like that. Are you stupid or incompetent? Or both? That's just fucking stupid. What are you going to do, kick me out of the network? Besides, have you read my contract? You don't realize you have been paying me for this service for twenty-eight years and I'm saving you money? I get $30 for an X-ray. You pay the hospital $260 for the film and $60 to read it. I do it all for $30.00!"

"Maybe—if we have to."

"Good luck with that. You've had a precedent set for all these decades, not even months or years, but decades, where I do my X-rays."

So the higherups sent a request for our quality assurance, qualifications, X-ray techs—reasonable questions. We answered all of them—what a hassle. Then AmeriHealth harasses me about infusions.

Let's say that a patient says, "I have lupus and I moved here from wherever; can you just refill my meds?"

I would say, "Well, if you are already on them, I'll continue them. But I need to do my due diligence to see if I agree with your diagnosis. Do you feel better than you did ten years ago when they started treating you?" If they say yes, then I'm more likely to agree. But I've had countless cases for which the diagnosis had been wrong for years and not only was the patient not improving but he or she didn't even know what was wrong!

Just recently, before I went into the room to see a patient, Denise, my medical assistant, said, "Doc, this woman is here for a second opinion. She has gone to a rheumatologist twenty miles north of here and has a label of rheumatoid arthritis, and the patient herself is skeptical. She wants a second opinion. The patient has scleroderma." This is my medical assistant telling me this. I walked in the room and talked to the lady, asking her a few questions. I looked at her blood. I said, "Ma'am, you have scleroderma, not rheumatoid arthritis."

She said, "Tell me: Why are you sure about that? Because the other doctor said my scleroderma test, when he repeated it, was only slightly above normal."

"Well, first of all, when I asked you if your hands were puffy, you said yes. That would be a distinctive feature of scleroderma. I asked you several other things that are more specific for scleroderma than other conditions. You said yes to those as well. Furthermore, two of the three rheumatoid arthritis tests were normal, and the third one wasn't done. But I can see that the first time you went to that guy your scleroderma antibody was thirty-five. Normal is less than twenty. He said that was really high, but he didn't understand why. He wanted to repeat it. He repeated it and a different lab did it. The result was

1.8. But the normal there was under 0.9." He explained to her that the 1.8 was so low that it wasn't important, and that meant she didn't have scleroderma.

"But," I said, "do you understand that 1.8 over 0.9 is a 100 percent increase while thirty-five over twenty is a 75 percent increase? The one where you were told it was barely over is actually more significant because it's higher, proportionally. Besides, you have all the features of scleroderma, and you are on methotrexate and you tell me you feel better? Yes. Okay, fine. Do you know that for the past seventy years, methotrexate has been used to reduce inflammatory joints?" Rheumatoid arthritis, scleroderma, myositis, lupus, Sjogren syndrome—those are the five connective-tissue diseases where you just give methotrexate and people at least feel better.

Then there is asymptomatic synovitis. Synovitis is the inflammation of the synovium. You can see it sometimes in the knuckles when the synovium is squishy. I said, "Ma'am, you might feel good, but you have very, very profound inflammatory synovitis. Methotrexate is not enough for you. Did you have a CAT scan of your lungs? Did you have an echocardiogram?"

"No," she said. "I didn't have any of that. Why are you asking?"

"Those are the basics in scleroderma because the leading cause of death is lung disease. You do have scleroderma, and you've never had any scleroderma evaluation and you feel better on methotrexate. That's it."

That's unbelievable, yet I see it all the time. So many people don't have a clue about what they are doing.

## What Is an Infusion?

What exactly is an infusion? An infusion is the administration of a liquid that, presumably, has beneficial medicine. When you go to the emergency room dehydrated, hospital workers hook up an IV and put up a bag of normal saline. That's an infusion. Some infusions take ten minutes. One particular product takes six or eight hours. By and large, most of the infusions I do take between twenty and ninety minutes, sometimes close to two hours. The common ones take a couple of hours, and they are administered about once every two months.

Let me break it down even further. Suppose during the examination of a patient I notice some swelling. I ask a few questions and get a blood test. I may even prescribe a strong anti-inflammatory drug for a few days. The blood test comes back and shows rheumatoid arthritis. Thirty-five years ago, rheumatoid arthritis left untreated was the "bad" arthritis. It was crippling. Now because we have these biologic drugs, we can reverse the course of the disease. Anybody with more than very mild disease goes on a biologic. (Remember, the biologics are medications that can't be made into pills because the molecules are too big, and they can't be in the stomach because the stomach acid will destroy them. They have to be given through a needle, either through the skin or into a vein. Delivery through the vein is better.)

Our rheumatoid arthritis patient will generally get a two-hour infusion every two months. For osteoporosis, the patient will get a subcutaneous injection every six months, or a ten-minute infusion once a year. It's all based on the half-life of the drug. These drugs completely revolutionized the field—they are incredibly effective. They were gamechangers, nuclear weapons.

An AmeriHealth rep said, "Wait a minute—you are not an accredited infusion center."

I said, "I never said I am an infusion center. I do in-office infusion."

"But you told Frank, and he saw for himself, that it operates like an infusion center."

"I could operate it like a pizza shop if I chose to," I said. "But it's still part of my office. If insurance doesn't cover pizza, I would understand it because it's not part of medical care. But again, you've been paying for infusions at my office just like DXA scans, X-rays, and me reading my synovial fluid, which is CLIA certified." (CLIA is the federal government certification for clinical labs.)

AmeriHealth *demanded*—with a five-day window—I either get accredited as an infusion site by one of the five or six accrediting agencies that it recognizes or I'd be terminated as a provider.

I told my CEO, "You know what, go ahead, get it. Because maybe we'll need it. Maybe in the future it will help us. It can't be bad to have it." Within five days, my CEO had vetted the companies and found out which one was best for us. One of them specializes in office infusion. Fine, I said. Let's do it. But it's clear it's all about making money. If my office signs up with Company X, it's $35,000 a year just to belong. The one we found is $2,000 a year, and it certifies offices that are doing infusions, something I've been doing for longer than the organization has been around.

But it gets better! My lawyer gets a letter from the accrediting agency. It's a full page: "Dr. Soloway's office, Arthritis, and Rheumatology Associates, is now enrolled in our program," and all the other things it needs to say.

My lawyers send it on within the time frame. The next day the lawyers from AmeriHealth called the accreditation company saying, "We are giving you six months, not twelve."

*Wait a minute*, I'm thinking. *You told us to pick somebody on this list. We did. You told us to prove that we're enrolled. We did. We picked somebody from your list, and they verified what you need to know. Now you are calling and questioning them that maybe we're still not qualified for all the laws? We follow the state laws first. I was a member of the Board of Medical Examiners; I know the New Jersey state laws better than they do. In the State of New Jersey, as long as I'm available by telephone, what we do is legal.* (The logic there is that if we have an emergency, we have to call 911. It's extremely rare, but it happens, and it's usually because an obese guy passes out because he didn't get a soda or something. It's not a drug-related issue. It's a slip and fall.)

The infusion accreditation company told AmeriHealth all of this. But the truth is, they're on a witch hunt. They saw the numbers, and thought, *Hey, we are spending too much money. This guy must be stealing. Let's go after him however we can.*

Well, little did they know, I'm the doc that says, "Fuck you! We're doing it my way, or your patients can't come here." Of course, I come from a leveraged position. "Where are you going to take your 150 people in the next three days? What are you going to do with them? You are going to tell them you can't go to the doctor?" I take that stance, and I've been on the winning side of every fight. But if I didn't fight for these patients, they'd be treated in a humdrum way. "You have arthritis, and that's just how you have to live now," they'd be told.

I've written several letters to AmeriHealth in response to its abhorrent treatment of patients. I'm including them in this book so that readers—patients and doctors—can see what is possible and what is effective. You can—and must—fight for proper treatment. Here is one from June 2021:

> TO: AmeriHealth Administrators Appeals Department
>
> RE: Diagnosis of large vessel vasculitis and request and denial for Rituximab.
>
> The above patient has life-threatening disease. Rituximab was requested and denied. The denial states that two non-preferred Rituximab similar drugs were not used. First, I have never been notified in writing or by phone call that there is such a policy set. Second, my office stocks the drug which the patient needs urgently. Third, no local facility or hospital stocks either biosimilar or Rituximab except mine. I am the only provider in Cumberland County who provides Rituximab, and this includes the hospital system. You indicate that the company designates these biosimilar products because there is no data for reliable evidence that any one brand of Rituxan is better than the other. That being said, we do know for certain that a person with life-threatening disease cannot wait for me to order other drugs, nor should the patient have to be subjected to such cruelty because of the parsimonious nature and egregious actions by your insurance company. It is further noted that while there is no evidence that Rituxan is better, there is also no evidence that biosimilars are equal or the same. Based on the grave nature of the patient's disease, in the time waiting merely to order another drug as a trial to appease your company she will end up being admitted to the

hospital, spending $200,000.00 compared to the cost of infusion in the office, which as you are aware is far cheaper than the infusion in the hospital.

I suggest this be overturned immediately before you have blood on your hands.

Sincerely,
Stephen Soloway, M.D.

These sorts of denials are so common that it is practically a full-time job fighting with the insurance companies over them. Here is another letter regarding a patient who was denied for Enbrel injections:

TO: AmeriHealth New Jersey Appeals Unit

I am in receipt of your deplorable letter regarding [Patient] and his denial for Enbrel injection. As you are probably unaware, [Patient] has been on Enbrel for his condition for more than ten years with good success. I find it obstructive, feckless, and churlish on the medical director's part, if he was even involved in the decision-making process, to deny such an inno-cent request. If somebody in your department has more knowledge on this topic than myself, I would suggest that person contact me or [Patient], who is a prominent attorney in his field. I expect you to overturn this immediately or I will see you in court.

Thank you in advance for your cooperation.

Stephen Soloway, M.D.

## Billing Codes

It's a constant, senseless, grinding fight with these companies. Remember, it's not just government overreach. It's government *and* corporate overreach. Corporate is both pharmaceutical and insurance: UnitedHealthcare,

Humana, Cigna, AmeriHealth, Independence Blue Cross, Blue Cross Blue Shield of New Jersey. It's all overreach because they all have something to say about how you treat your patients, and none of them can do a fraction of what I can do.

I actually had a good relationship with the CEO of one of the Horizon companies for many years before he quit his job. I know that insurance companies are always looking to save money. So I made him an offer years ago. Codes are used in billing: 1, 2, 3, 4, 5, and so on. Code 1 may be the least complicated and 5 the most complicated, the longest, the most expensive. Code 1 is the nurse only, and 2 is you walk in the room, and you walk out. Let's say 3 and 4 are the two main billing codes. I said to the CEO, "Why don't you take the average of what you pay me for 3 and 4, come up with one price, and make it the same for both? You don't have to order 3s and 4s. And you can say there is no financial motivation for me to put 4s."

He said, "That's a great idea." For that company, my 3s and 4s are the same amounts of money. And the truth is, we don't make our money on a $50 or $60 visit. It's completely irrelevant. But if we want to give the perception that we don't give a shit, that's one way to do it. Now they don't audit me for this stuff. They don't look because I can't be billing 4s all the time and be motivated financially since I get paid the same for high- and low-level visits.

He actually told me at one point, "We audited you so many times. We didn't come up with anything. You are a solid guy. You are a good guy. We don't have patient complaints. We don't have anything to complain about."

I said, "That's because my patients are infused and don't do self-injectables. My patients are not being admitted to the hospital. When I go to the hospital to see a patient, that patient is never one of mine." Another rheumatologist from another town has the patient, who is just not being treated aggressively or watched closely enough.

"Here we have forced compliance," I said, "and it works. Furthermore, the infusible drugs—and nobody believes this—in the office setting are cheaper than the home self-injectables."

Not a week after we received the letter about AmeriHealth, I was notified by the Humana insurance company that I had to be certified to read my X-rays, even though, again, I have been reading them myself for the past *thirty years* and I have two certified X-ray techs. That's the exact same problem! How stupid are these people?

Humana claimed I was not qualified to read X-rays because I'm not an orthopedic surgeon. Since when did orthopedic surgeons read rheumatologic X-rays?

Around the same time, I had almost the same issue with Burns company, which also insisted my office become certified as an infusion center. Because I am so large, they will not accept that I am just an office. But that's the truth. What I do in the office is all legal, but the insurance companies will not allow it. So against state and all other law, they decide what they like or don't like. Now they don't like me doing infusions despite the fact that it's great forced compliance, the prices are the lowest, and they are cheaper than self-injectable drugs. However, they've decided that since I expanded my office, my enlargement or expansion is not part of my office, and they want me to be accredited by the Joint Commission on Accreditation of Healthcare Organizations (JCAHO), which is $25,000 a year and no benefit whatsoever. However, if I followed their rules, the patients would be screwed, and the insurance company would lose money. The people working in decision-making positions at insurance companies may be at a high intellectual latitude. However, 99 percent of the people below them are somewhere underwater.

In the past, all insurance companies would furnish a provider representative to service the account, which would be the medical facility or medical practice. The account representative would either have a zip code or hospitals or private offices or a mix of things. There are no representatives anymore. I have no one to call, no one to discuss problems with. So what can I do but write vicious letters to CEOs and upper-level management and occasionally hire private investigators to get us their actual phone numbers and addresses so that I can direct patients to their homes? It is just a method of waking them up!

Our political leaders are helpful, but they are less helpful when it comes to private insurance companies, as they claim the ability to legally assist with the government plans (ironic and hypocritical). That seems to be the end of the government's ability to interfere in private healthcare. I don't understand why, as it interferes in all other private sectors by overregulating. Medicare and Medicaid are so overregulated that the right and the left never know what is going on.

The lengths the insurance companies will go to in order to make illogical, stupid, and harmful decisions are extraordinary. Not long ago, I received a letter from Aetna stating that it contacted my patients that receive biologic infusion at my office and encouraged them to have it done at home. The letter also said that I should encourage patients to receive the infusion at home.

This is quite disingenuous. It is more expensive to have it done at home than it is in the office.

If I am going to discuss nonmedical issues, I am wasting my time and the patient's time. If I were taking patients from my office, where there is guaranteed compliance and lower cost, I would be doing a disservice to the patient and the system. Let's say I have fifty patients, and let's just pretend each patient represents $1,000. Well, if you take them out of my practice, and you send them to home infusion, now they become a $1,200 burden on society. Plus you are going to piss me off. Maybe I'm going to start to order extra testing. Finally, based on Aetna's suggestion that I speak to my patients under Aetna about why the change would be better for them, I figured maybe what is better is discussing the option of a different insurance company.

I couldn't believe what they were doing. I wrote the following letter in response:

To: Karen Lynch, CEO, CVS Health Aetna

With dismay and shock I received a letter indicating you have reached out to my patients having infusion of biologic drugs, and the advice that I should discuss with them home infusion as you suggest. The patients all receive infusion at my office which is 10% cheaper than home infusion. In case you are not aware of this, wake up. You are under the assumption that people infused from my practice are getting done at the hospital, where it is 50%-65% more expensive. If you are not aware of this, wake up, and do not send such ridiculous letters in the future.

Further, if you think I have time to discuss anything other than healthcare problems with your patients, I don't. The only discussion I would have with them are the benefits of insurances and pharmacies other than the ones they currently have. Hopefully you can read between the lines. I am not a feckless curmudgeon, and I do not take nonsense lightly. This whisper campaign must cease and desist immediately, or unpredictable consequences will ensue.

Please be guided accordingly.

Stephen Soloway, M.D.

Talk about unethical: the insurance company owns the home infusion company! Under no circumstances should Aetna be reaching out to my patients.

You have to educate your patients. In my office, I'm the cheapest, and I'm the most convenient. If you go to a hospital, you have to drive to the hospital, park, walk a thousand feet, talk to some TSA agent who asks you a bunch of questions. You have to sign in, and you are sent to the ninth floor. When you get there, you have to show your ID, sign in, fill out the forms.

In my office—and in any good office—workers know you. They have your infusion ready. You are in and out.

The patients know me; I diagnosed them. They are ecstatic that I helped them when nobody else did. They don't want to go anywhere else, least of all to home infusion!

I can't be the only doctor that has this sort of clout. But when you have tens of thousands of patients, and you are the only one in an area, I do. I am the rainmaker! Aetna told my lawyer that it was going to terminate my contract. But it can't, not with the number of patients I see. I'd simply see their patients without network benefits, and they'd end up paying me more.

These companies try to browbeat everybody! They can't browbeat me. I don't need them.

For good measure, here is a letter I wrote to the CEO of Aetna Better Health New Jersey in response to Aetna reaching out to a patient in an effort to get that person to stop seeing me:

---

TO: Glenn A. MacFarlane, CEO, Aetna Better Health NJ

The patient above was approached via telephone by Aetna Better Health who suggested the patient stop seeing Dr. Soloway. They browbeat her. She insisted she wanted to stay with New Jersey Horizon NJ Health (because of Dr. Soloway).

This is one of the most outrageous, complicit, egregious, and incorrigible jokes that no patient should have to deal with. No patient should be browbeaten by an insurance company to switch for their financial benefit. No patient should be encouraged to switch a doctor who is helping them. I am a specialist serving the southern 12 counties in New Jersey. I am a rarity in my field, taking all insurance. I will not allow these types of games to be played.

One should note, Aetna Health Plans has taken away provider relation coordinators, and physicians treating Aetna patients have no contact person. The only way to get their attention would be to cease and desist from seeing their patients and let their patients complain and write letters to Mr. MacFarlane, the CEO of Aetna Better Health NJ.

If a patient with insurance can receive healthcare and is browbeat by another company for financial benefit, this is a criminal act. This action will not be taken lightly. Please have your legal department advise. Please be aware that this action will be taken to the Division of Banking and Insurance State of New Jersey, Congress United States of America, private attorney and legal firms, and the State Board of Medical Examiners. Please note that I am a Fellow of the Federation of State Medical Boards. Your time is running out and my patience is done.

Sincerely,
Stephen Soloway, M.D.

# CHAPTER 6
# FIGHTING FOR MY PATIENTS

## Why I Fight For My Patients

Sometimes I fight insurance companies for my office or my practice. But more often I'm fighting for patients, who do not know how to fight for themselves and who, frankly, don't have the leverage that I do.

Most doctors don't know they can write letters or who to send them to. Most don't know what to say—I don't know why, because I do. But I can tell you, if you are employed by a hospital, you just follow directions and move along. You don't cause any trouble; you don't say a word. And the care shows.

I'm the anomaly—a doctor who gives a shit—which is why my success rate and patient satisfaction is unheard of. Of course, it's also why the FBI has been investigating me for five years. They wonder how I can possibly do all this work. Nobody ever asks why my patients don't get admitted to the hospital. How does he work so efficiently? Why does he have so many accolades and so few complaints? Why do his patients wait for hours and days? If big government has anything to do with your reimbursement, simply stated, you are fucked.

The answer is because I force them to do things correctly, which they do. I'm *saving* the system money because I keep the people out of the hospital. I don't order unnecessary tests, imaging, or surgery.

Fighting for patients makes me ten steps better than everyone else because my patients actually get better while the other people's patients die. But I don't just want to be good at what I do. I want to be the best. I enjoy being the best. You can't be the best if you don't offer every service. That includes fighting with insurance companies for the patient.

I've written some brutally nasty, personal notes to some high-ranking people at these companies. I just don't give a shit. I want them out there, which is why I am including them in this book. I'm not looking to make enemies, but I want people to see how hard you have to fight.

I need to fight for my patients, and patients need to fight for themselves because a war is going on. The insurance companies need to preserve their income, and to do so, they deny everything. What am I going to do? I could tell the patient, "I'm sorry, your company is not paying. Your insurance sucks." Or I can fight the insurance. I also tell the patients to call to make a complaint and tell the insurance company they are going to switch companies.

People don't know to do this. I've had patients tell me they couldn't come to me for a year because they couldn't get a referral. I tell them they don't need a referral.

"Really?" they say, "The doctor said I needed one."

I say, "The doctor didn't want you to come to me because he's jealous of me."

I saw a patient the other day who was having a bad flare because his insurance changed. He was told there was a three-month grace in the change, but his medication was stopped because nobody would pay for it. His new insurance coverage, a combination of Medicare and Cigna, would not approve the drug he was previously taking. Cigna, which is the secondary coverage, has decided that the patient could not be on the drug because it is not on the formulary.

To compound the issue, the drug Cigna would not pay for is the *least expensive* drug in its class! This is illegal and yet it occurs all the time.

The first thing I do when I hear of a situation like this is write a horrific, nasty letter. If the companies don't want to get involved, or they don't help, I reach out to the congressman's office: "You have to get on this for me now." That's what happens when you donate to politicians!

I just sent a letter threatening to sue Aetna if it doesn't pay a bill. It caved. You have to have leverage, otherwise you are sure to fail.

I love being able to say, "No, if you don't let me use the drug I want to use then go fuck yourself. Your patient will not be seen here. Next I'm going to send them to your house, and you can explain why you are not allowing their drug to be paid for."

Let's look at the situation of a patient I have named Mario, who happens to be the son of my assistant, Carleen. Here is Mario's story in Carleen's words:

My son, who is thirty-four years old, has had numerous stomach problems and pain in his legs. He went to doctor after doctor after doctor. He went to specialist after specialist. And they all said, "We don't really see anything wrong with you. Your bloodwork is coming out. We think you just have a hernia. But your hernia is too small right now to even operate."

So I said to my son, "I want you to come see Dr. Soloway. Give it a shot. Just talk to Dr. Soloway. See what he says." So my son came in. Dr. Soloway did what he does with all new patients. He spoke with him and asked questions while touching various joints and skin. He ordered tons of blood tests. They must have taken twenty-five vials of blood! But on that first visit, Dr. Soloway looked at my son and said, "You have Crohn's disease, and you have ankylosing spondylitis. But let's take these tests and let's confirm what I have to say. In the meantime, I want you to take this medicine."

When the tests came in, my son came back and Dr. Soloway said, "Yep, you have Crohn's and the ankylosing spondylitis. What I want you to do is to start Remicade." My son did three months of Remicade, and the kid was awesome. He said, "Mom, I feel like I have my life back. I feel like a brand-new person."

The next thing we know I come home from work, and he says "Mom, they denied my Remicade. The insurance company denied my Remicade because they want me to try this other medicine instead. I have to go on

*(Continued on next page)*

this medicine for the next couple treatments. If that doesn't work, then maybe I can go back on Remicade, or we'll find another medicine."

Of course, Dr. Soloway got the letter, too, and he was furious.

When it came time for his next infusion, my son didn't know what to do. But he went and got it, and he got deathly ill from this other medication. He was out of work for over a week with terrible pains in his stomach. He said to me, "I'm never doing this again. I'm not going to go back and get this medicine. It makes me sick. I can't lose work."

So Dr. Soloway started writing letters on my son's behalf. He just kept writing letters and writing letters telling the insurance company that my son was doing well on Remicade, and they've made him sick again. He didn't give up.

And my son refused to get an infusion of the other medicine. So I guess they finally saw he wasn't going, and they weren't getting paid, so they approved his Remicade. He got an infusion, and now he's fine.

The insurance companies just assume people will not fight. You can even hear other doctors say, "Really, you can do that? We didn't know we could do that." But you have to fight them for yourself and on behalf of patients.

It is just absolutely amazing. The insurance companies are not the doctor. When did the insurance companies become doctors? If they wanted to be doctors, then they should have gotten the degree.

I've known Dr. Soloway for about twenty years. I was a patient before I started working for him. I had neck issues, and the first time that I met Dr. Soloway, as a patient, I only had about an hour wait, which was pretty remarkable compared to how it is now. But he was very thorough—a lot of testing, X-rays, DXA scans, MRIs. He figured it out right away. I knew of his reputation from friends. And we had met a couple times through political events as well. I happened to be the vice chair of the Cumberland County Republican Association. And obviously he was a donor.

When I became his personal assistant, it was an eye-opener for me. What the insurance companies are doing to patients and to doctors is absolutely atrocious. The denial letters come in every day. And these letters are ridiculous. That's where I go into PubMed or whatever research I can do to tell them, "No, you are wrong. This is what the patient needs. These are the medical articles, medical journals, and case studies that all prove that this is the right medication." It's just amazing how the insurance companies operate, and it's all for money. They've lost their way. Everything is about money. It's not about the original goal—to make patients better. That was the biggest wake-up call that I had.

So that's how it goes. Mario had been taking Remicade for a while and was 100 percent better. The insurance company made a unilateral decision that he needs to be on a different medication. The insurance company's choice was a substitute—a biosimilar—and the reason for it was to save the insurance company money. I wrote a letter to the COO of Meritain Health:

TO: Meritain Health

I find myself in a very disturbed position. This patient has a clinical diagnosis of Crohn's disease, and to control his abdominal pain and joint symptoms he is taking biologic therapy. His endoscopy was approved and scheduled and at the last minute cancelled by his insurance company. This occurred the week of June 20th. He missed a week of work in preparation for testing, had Covid test with 72-hour quarantine, and then endoscopy was canceled on June 23rd. This, the third time the patient has had similar circumstances, being told the week of May 2nd and May 23rd

*(Continued on next page)*

that he had approval for testing (MRI and endoscopy), taking the week off of work for Covid and quarantine, and then having the approval canceled at the last minute.

I find it outrageous, egregious, and complicit to have a patient told at the last minute after missing work and preparing for a procedure that it is their responsibility to have the procedure at a "cheaper location." That said, insurance companies must negotiate better terms with hospitals.

This deplorable situation should be the start for a greater dialogue; however, we have cost a man work and wasted time, angst, anguish, despair, and most importantly no definitive diagnosis. If this were your family, would this be acceptable to you?

Sincerely,
Stephen Soloway, M.D.

Less than a year later, I had to write to the company again:

TO: Meritain Health

With dismay, your company does not allow "buy and bill" for biologic drugs. To make it worse, the drugs I prescribe to patients are not accepted by your formulary. I am prepared to delete you from my network; you do not meet my quality standards. I advise you I am the only full-time rheumatology practice in this county. I recommend you think about this dilemma and have senior management meet me immediately at my convenience. I will personally discuss this with your patients, and I will show them available insurance companies and let them decide which is in their best interest.

I cite one example: Patient Mario on Remicade 100% better; you changed his drug to save money. He is no longer able to contribute to society. I fixed him after many years of delayed diagnosis.

Remicade is the least expensive TNF inhibitor. Either you are receiving kickbacks and rebates, or you are just plain ultracrepidarians.

Thank you for your anticipated cooperation.

Sincerely,
Stephen Soloway, M.D.

Several months later, I was still fighting:

TO: Meritain Health

The patient has Crohn's colitis and had 100% sensitive response to Remicade. He has had 3 Remicade infusions. Your company has denied continued use of Remicade. Your company has insisted on failure of Inflectra first. The patient has already been on Remicade. State law prohibits changing for no reason. Further, switching and then trying to go back in the future causes increased immunogenicity and more likely that the drug will not work. Remicade, not Remicade-like drugs, is the best product. Remicade is the same price when administered in the office as Inflectra. There is no reason at all to torture this patient. If this were your brother, I would hope that you would provide better care, knowing that cost is not being sacrificed.

If this is not overturned immediately, this patient will with my assistance, have immediate legal support, private and public. In addition, I will cease immediately to see any patients with your insurance.

Sincerely,
Stephen Soloway, M.D.

And I *will* cease to see the patients. I'll have them call this asshole and bombard her.

I've done that with UnitedHealthcare in the past. I will do it again if I need to.

After I sent the last letter, I received a call from the senior business research analyst/provider from the insurance company trying to help solve the problem. I found out a specialty pharmacy subcontracted by Meritain Health handled this situation, not the insurance company. Apparently, the pharmacy benefits manager (PBM) made the change based on its financial needs at the time. It wants the lowest-cost drug whether it is good or bad; however, the lowest-cost drug is essentially not less expensive than the drug I was using. As alternatives have come along, the price of Remicade has gone down.

In my vast experience, Remicade is a better drug. Data supports it is likely the best in its class for many conditions. The specialty pharmacy, acting like a battery-operated robot, went against doctor's orders and against the policy of the insurance company for which it works. The lesson here is not to switch a medicine that is working! Nobody should be taking an inferior product.

What is unusual is that the pharmacy approved the drug Aria, which is two-and-a-half times the price of Remicade.

I wrote a separate letter to Meritain Health regarding its denials:

---

TO: Meritain Health

Ladies and Gentlemen:

This letter is in reference to the 20 active patients of yours that I am currently treating. I am a board-certified rheumatologist four times over, and I also maintain my boards in internal medicine. I am a White House appointee and an honorary member of the Federation of State Medical Boards. I take patient care very seriously. With unprecedented authority you have been denying my patients access to Remicade. It is unfounded to change a patient to a medication for the benefit of saving $5 per vial, yes

$5 per vial. If you were one of my patients, you would not wish this type of horrible care or treatment from an insurance company on yourself.

This deplorable behavior will not be tolerated at Arthritis and Rheumatology Associates of South Jersey. We are the leaders in the area. We have the most Top Doctor awards. I am the Chairman of Rheumatology of the entire Inspira Health System including Vineland, Elmer, and Mullica Hill campuses. My practice does not and will not stock more medication than is necessary. I will not be using Inflectra on your patients, and if one has slipped through the cracks they will be changed. You should know that Aria, also known as Simponi Aria, is far more expensive, yet it is a first-tier drug with your company. Inflectra and Remicade are the same price. The differential is less than $5 per vial.

You can feel free to reach out by telephone as letters take too long to discuss this issue, but I will not be using biosimilar medications merely because you tell me to. This is a non-starter and I wished to tell you this in writing. I will dictate what drugs the patients get in my practice. I will also dictate what the formulary is at this practice. Further attempts to sabotage the care of the patients will be met with very stern actions.

Sincerely,
Stephen Soloway, M.D.

---

Meritain or Cigna or Blue Cross doesn't do this alone. All of them do. They are all motivated by the same thing, and it isn't the patient's health! At this very moment, for example, Aetna Healthcare is also refusing to pay for Remicade for two of my patients.

The two patients are stable and have been on the same drug for the last ten years. Aetna, as I've discussed, has been engaged in a very loud whisper campaign. It has contacted all of my patients on Remicade and told them to discuss with me going on home infusion, which costs 10 percent more than the office infusion. In addition, coincidentally, Aetna and CVS have teamed up and are now one company. It wants full control over patient medication and does not allow choices. It has a preferred list and secondary list. On the secondary list are drugs it doesn't want on the primary list. Interestingly, the patients who are told they must switch off Remicade, which helps them, are given no option. First-tier drugs are preferred and presumably are chosen due to the cost. Second-tier drugs are far more expensive, due to the administration at the hospital. The office infusion is the cheapest option, even cheaper than self-injectable drugs. These people are too stupid to understand that infusions are more expensive in a hospital and my practice is not a hospital.

Sadly, Aetna has been asking patients to come off Remicade, have the procedure done at home, or use self-injectables or another in the same class, which is double the price.

I wrote two letters to the CEO about this:

TO: Karen Lynch CEO CVS Health Aetna

Today, I was to have a peer-to-peer review scheduled at 11:30 a.m. EST with Richard Robinson, a clinical pharmacist. Mr. Robinson told my nurse Carleen that there was no reason to speak to me since he would not overturn his decision. He offered another phone number that I can call to get another peer-to-peer with somebody else in 72 hours or less perhaps. You are jeopardizing the life and the treatment of patients who are currently working. If you stop their Remicade or don't allow them to be treated, for in this patient's case relapsing polychondritis, the patient will die. If the patient dies, that will be your fault. I previously submitted many articles documenting the use of Remicade in relapsing polychondritis. This is an extremely rare disease. There are no drugs indicated to treat except Prednisone. Standard of care states if the patient fails Prednisone next step up is Remicade. If the patient cannot tolerate steroids—use Remicade.

While there are not enough patients to conduct randomized control trials with this disease and this drug, there was a clear consensus that the standard of care indicates this drug works, and I have submitted the articles previously and had a preemptive denial on a phone call with a subordinate for a peer-to-peer call.

Not all diseases are treated with Prednisone alone. Not all rare diseases have specific medications indicated. I provided enough articles, and the patient does not have time to wait. If necessary, I will administer drugs without an authorization number and I will charge you double.

Sincerely,

Stephen Soloway, M.D.

TO: Karen Lynch CEO CVS Health Aetna

Dear Ms. Lynch:

I wrote due to the following behavior. It is incorrigible, suspicious, complicit, and nefarious. We receive blanket denials for Remicade patients that are stable with the drug for 10 plus years. You are not aware of this. Remicade has immunogenicity. You stop the drug, you restart, and it doesn't work. People will not be stopping the drug. You will be subjected to civil and criminal litigation. Your leftist despot ideology will not be tolerated in this practice. As you are aware, an orthopedic group left your insurance company in my area. You paid a lot more for out-of-network benefits. Their practice is dwarfed by the behemoth that I have. Your job is to sell insurance and honor the policies. Your job is not to be a financial controller.

When the Aetna patients ask why they cannot be seen at this office, the answer will be simple; I am too busy writing letters to people who steal

*(Continued on next page)*

your money. Here at Arthritis and Rheumatology we provide the patients with all information including the names, addresses, and phone numbers of CEOs, medical directors, and everyone else involved in the hindrance of their care. If you think anyone cares about protecting your freedoms and rights, if they are not doing it for the Supreme Court Justices they really don't give a shit about you.

I will only deal with upper-level management. Peer-to-peer is ridiculous. You do not have any peers in rheumatology. Peer-to-peer would be CEO to CEO, and your decisions are not medical; they are financial only. If you choose to make financial decisions, then we will have a peer-to-peer, and it will be a peer-to-peer; it will not be a dictating session to me.

I hope to hear from the management team as I have in the past. I refer you back two weeks when I wrote the same letter and had two other patients in the same situation overturned, [Patient] and [Patient]. It is your job to overturn or fix your broken policies that are leading to my wasted time, as I will waste my time when it comes to your patients who will then go out of network, and you will have to pay me double. I have all the answers on how to save everyone money and provide proper care. This is something that no one else understands. Perhaps reading my 25-page CV solely in private practice will shed some light on my superior intelligence.

Sincerely,

Stephen Soloway, M.D.

While enraging, I do not accept the practice of insurance companies deciding unilaterally to switch patients from drugs that have worked for years, to save a few bucks, and I fight tooth and nail to get my patients the best product. If patients pay for insurance and I provide a service, my job is to not worry about how much money an insurance company spends. The front line soldier, the doctor, should be protected and paid very well while the insurance company and the government keep the crumbs, not the opposite. The following are two letters I sent to Aetna regarding a patient whose medication was cut off by his insurance company:

TO: Walter C. Wengel, III, Director of Physician Operations, Aetna Health Inc.

Dear Mr. Wengel:

This patient has severe tophaceous gout in a polyarticular distribution. This patient was appropriately given Krystexxa/Pegloticase after failure of conventional therapy. Based on severe disease and severe tophus burden, I opted to give him Krystexxa. The patient indicated to me for the first time in his life that he finally found a drug that was working for him. His tophus burden is visibly decreased in the hands, wrists, elbows, shoulders, hips, knees, ankles, metatarsals, and any nodules that he had.

The patient came in today very angry. Initially I thought his anger was directed at me. In fact, his anger is directed at Aetna Insurance Company. The patient has an Aetna plan and apparently was approved for twelve months of Krystexxa. Unbeknownst to him or me, his Krystexxa was cut off after three months. The patient will likely need treatment for anywhere from six to twelve months. I will give you the benefit of the doubt that perhaps this is an oversight and perhaps he needed to come in for a follow-up that required this letter. But if this is not sorted out in a very timely fashion, the patient and I will personally sue you to the fullest extent of the law as you are interfering with his healthcare.

Do not take this as an idle threat. I will go directly to Mark Bertolini, the CEO of your company, and have the State Insurance Commissioner and State Attorney General assist. This is a very serious matter, and this patient cannot live without Krystexxa. I expect he will be on it for six to twelve months or longer, and I expect this decision and/or problem to be fixed and/or overturned immediately if not sooner.

Sincerely yours,
Stephen Soloway, M.D.

To: Walter C. Wengel, III, Director of Physician Operations, Aetna Health Inc.

Mark T. Bertolini, Chief Executive Officer, Aetna Health Inc.

Gentlemen:

At an alarming rate, I am having disturbing results dealing with Aetna Insurance Company.

To cut to the chase:

[Patient] was approved for Krystexxa (Pegloticase) for twelve months. After three infusions, his insurance cut him off. His insurance was Aetna Health. This is unprecedented and has no basis. The patient needs this drug, and the patient is doing well on this drug. He has no side effects. The patient fulfilled all criteria to get the drug. This is a difficult patient. He needs six to twelve months to be debulked with respect to his tophus burden. I am an expert in the field, a published author, and this is unacceptable.

Patients on biologic therapy such as Remicade (Infliximab). Using Remicade as an example, be advised Remicade 5 mg/kg every six weeks is the starting dose for ankylosing spondylitis, 40% more than the rheumatoid arthritis dose, and is 50% less expensive than any self-injectable rheumatoid product. Hence, my next statement.

Your patients are being denied this drug if more than 600 mg for psoriatic arthritis is used. I can justify this as quite ridiculous by virtue that the drug is dosed by weight. And if an overweight person cannot even get their starting dose because of the Aetna guidelines, there is a serious problem within the Aetna Health System.

I have reached out to Mr. Bertolini on various occasions via telephone and seem to get nowhere. Mr. Wengel has become more difficult to reach as time goes on and a year or so ago advised that he would be my representative as my field rep is frankly an obnoxious witch. I prefer to deal with upper-level management as I too am a CEO of a company. The company is Arthritis & Rheumatology Associates of SJ, the most prestigious and largest solo Rheumatology practice in the United States of America. We do everything right. We offer all services under one roof. We make everything convenient for patients. We do not overcharge. We do not overbill. We do not overtreat. We do not overmedicate.

What you are doing to your patients is simply amoral. If these disingenuous actions do not cease, I will stop at nothing within the legal system to make things right. I trust we will have in-person communication or, worst-case scenario, telephone communication within the next ten business days. Kindly be advised accordingly, I anxiously await communication amongst us. This is the tip of the iceberg and needs to be quashed immediately.

Thank you for your anticipated cooperation.


Sincerely yours,

Stephen Soloway, M.D.

---

Next is a critically ill young lupus patient with concurrent vasculitis:

---

TO: Mark Bertolini

CC: Congressman Jeff Van Drew

Dear Mark,

Read below:

[The] 23-year-old female with a full life to live has a grave picture painted in my note. The deficiencies in your insurance company are so wide Russian tanks could drive through. If this were your daughter or granddaughter, I would hope you have a better judgment and attitude about what testing

(Continued on next page)

should be done. I have no interest in knowing what money I am saving or costing the insurance company. I am only interested in how I benefit patients with the best technical testing available. Failure to allow proper testing could wind up in the death of the patient. I and the patient's mother will hold you personally accountable if this is not changed immediately.

Stephen Soloway, M.D.

Apparently the company is too wrapped up in guidelines but not standards of care, and we already know how I feel about guidelines. In the case of this next letter, the company wanted a stepwise approach. But a stepwise approach is not wise. Early aggressive treatment was needed.

TO: Aetna Better Health of New Jersey Appeal and Grievance Department

To Whom It May Concern:

The policies implemented by your pharmacy benefit plan are not compatible with the standard of care. Patients with rheumatoid arthritis or spondyloarthropathies are not required to fail methotrexate for three months prior to starting a biologic agent; in fact it is the opposite. Early use of biologic DMARDs has been proven to be a benefit in these patients. Failure to comply with my policy, and I would consider myself the venerable and most senior and decorated rheumatologist in Philadelphia and South Jersey, will be met with my canceling my contract with your company. There is really nothing further to add except you are impeding the proper care of patients. As I have agreed to take Aetna Better Care at a lower rate and lose money, you too will need to take a loss and do what is right by the patient, not by your bank account. Do not feel castigated, I am merely stating the facts.

Sincerely,

Stephen Soloway, M.D.

This next patient needed this particular drug due to its inherent ability to influence whether a patient gets gout. Adherence to the formulary would be negligence to the patient. Family pets could do a better job:

---

RE: Walgreen Drug Change Request

The request for change on Losartan 100 mg is denied. I will not be forced to make alternative choices to save you money. The only way I can discuss changing medication would be for the company CEO to meet with me either virtual or in person. I am sure if you were the patient, you would understand my tenacity in helping my patients. A patient should receive the proper care, not what financially benefits the Walgreen formulary.

Thank you very much.


Stephen Soloway, M.D.

---

Next is a simple case of a company trying to save money. The requested drug has life-saving benefits, and although it is expensive, the company, Horizon in this case, has a code to pay for the product, and we accept its rate. Proper care is being prohibited here. If I wanted to waste money, I would use this drug on everybody:

---

TO: Sam Currie, Director, Pharmacy Services, Horizon BCBSNJ

EJ Blair, Director, Network Management Government Programs, Horizon BCBSNJ

RE: Rituximab denial

As you are aware, this patient needs Rituximab. Rituximab is not widely used in my practice. For the handful of patients that are on Rituximab, we stock Rituximab. I think I have been quite cooperative in the past, and for

*(Continued on next page)*

the one or two new starts of Rituximab. Please honor this request. I do not stock biosimilar of Rituximab on hand. We had a great working relationship in the past. I have done my part and am already saving you a tremendous sum of money. Please consider not holding up the Rituximab patients as they are few and far between. These patients are quite ill which is why I am using that drug first-line and they have far more problems than rheumatoid arthritis. They have immune neuropathy and a list of problems that are far more than a TNF can handle, therefore my choice of B cell depletion.

I hope you are both well and I look forward to a favorable response for this patient as soon as possible.

Sincerely,
Stephen Soloway M.D.

Sadly this insurance company is also not aware that two drugs indicated for lupus have different purposes.

TO: Horizon NJ Health

Answer to question: Why is member on both Benlysta and Lupkynis?

[Patient] has Class IV lupus nephritis. She has been treated for two years, and after two years her protein has come down from 30 grams to half a gram. Half a gram is a great start. However, normal is less than 150 mg. Plaquenil or hydroxychloroquine, and Benlysta or belimumab are the standard of care in lupus patients today as hydroxychloroquine as this patient is on has been proven to prevent lupus flare and hyperlipidemia and thrombus in lupus patients.

Benlysta has been proven to prevent organ damage in lupus. It is not specific for the kidneys. Lupkynis, a novel drug which is an interferon inhibitor, is specifically directed at skin and kidney in lupus. The

TULIP-2 trial indicates this is the case and there is no evidence to suggest that those drugs should not be given together. Furthermore, on a technicality, it would be more dangerous in theory to combine Benlysta and Rituximab which is commonly done in lupus nephritis patients. In fact, for a period of time this patient was on a combination of Benlysta and Rituximab, and studies have shown safety combining Benlysta and cyclophosphamide.

I have discussed this case at length with Michelle Petri, Director of Lupus at Johns Hopkins University. She is considered the world's leader and expert in the field of lupus. Lupkynis, a rather new approval, has shown great success thus far, and not using it is against the current standard of care for a patient with severe and chronic renal disease.

For another patient, I wrote a letter to appeal the insurance company's denial of Xanax:

TO: Prescription Claims Appeals MC 109-CVS Caremark

On behalf of [patient] who is a complicated lupus patient who I have treated for 25 years. [Patient] suffers from anxiety, depression, and headaches in addition to life-threatening hemolytic anemia, renal disease, liver disease, and other conditions. He has taken branded Xanax up to 10 years or more. He does well with this drug. Your formulary alternatives only offer generic benzodiazepines. You would not be aware that benzodiazepines work on threshold effect; hence generics, which have slightly less product—which is allowable under the law—would probably put him under his threshold and therefore the dose would be raised, the drug would be changed, and response would be different.

There is no logical rationale for changing one stable medicine for years. He is one of the few patients who I treat with benzodiazepines.

*(Continued on next page)*

What I note is that after all these years there is no tolerance or dependence. He merely takes it and does well. We are not going to change this now. Your denial is unfounded, and it is merely a financial denial and not a medical-based denial. Further, there has been trial and failure of Klonopin and Valium more than 20 years ago, and they merely did not work for him.

Enough with the game playing. The only valid explanation for denying the patients: they do not pay for their insurance or their bill. I trust you to figure this one out all by yourself and handle this.

Sincerely,
Stephen Soloway, M.D.

# CHAPTER 7
# THE "PEER-TO-PEER," PREAUTHORIZATION, AND MORE INSURANCE INCOMPETENCE

## What's the Backstory?

What's the backstory? The known "facts" are obviously inaccurate. What's really going on? Who's paying off whom? Who's getting a rebate, a kickback? Who is getting something to make it so that the more expensive drug is preferred over a drug that's half the price and better? A backstory tells the truth; one just has to know where to look.

Another patient of mine had been approved for Remicade on another insurance and got switched to a new insurance, which wanted to deny the Remicade because it's not on its formulary. Drugs are approved or denied at random. People's insurance switches, and a drug they've been on for years is no longer approved. This type of thing is criminal and pervasive.

So I write more letters. Here is one regarding a chronic asthma patient whose medication, Fasenra, was denied:

---

TO: OptumHealthCare Solutions LLC

RE: Fasenra denial

Fasenra (benralizumab) is an interlukin-5 inhibitor. This class of drug is to treat refractory asthma and other conditions with elevated mast cell activation, production, and elevated IgE levels. It is my oath to treat patients properly. Your responsibility is to facilitate this. This patient has chronic asthma, which is severe and not maintained on multiple

*(Continued on next page)*

---

treatments, currently short of breath with Ventolin 90 milliequivalents per actuation aerosol inhaler, and ipratropium, and has been on numerous other inhalers over the years, both in combination or alone. The patient has been on and had adverse reactions to Spiriva and Symbicort. The next step in treatment is either Xolair, which blocks eosinophils and is revolutionary in asthma, or the interleukin-5 inhibitors; without this the patient will require chronic steroids.

I am tired of writing letters to have approval of drugs that are necessary in patients who have insurance. The despotic power of the insurance companies is financially motivated and to not pay claims or allow patient access to what are deemed expensive drugs will not be tolerated by myself or the practice of Arthritis and Rheumatology Associates of South Jersey. I am well credentialed as a member of the Federation of State Medical Boards, the Chairman of the PEC, NJ Board of Medical Examiners, and an appointee of the President of the United States Council on Sports, Fitness, and Nutrition.

The best doctors do not follow guidelines. They understand guidelines are the basic lowest level of knowledge to practice medicine and start learning. Guidelines do not provide standard of care; they are merely a crutch for big insurance to prevent patients from obtaining proper medication if the medication is not in the budget.

Writing letters each time I need approval for medication will not be tolerated any longer. If necessary, I will employ the following actions if these denials continue and this patient mentioned is not approved: Newspapers and news outlets will be contacted, myself with the assistance of Senators and Congressmen will petition the main headquarters of your company, and/or I will reserve the right to withdraw from treating your patients.

I have been listed in Philadelphia Magazine for being the best in my field longer than any physician ever and remain current at 20 consecutive years. This letter is not meant to be frightening, but to alert you. If patients

> are treated, they are to be treated correctly. If not, they will all be switching insurance companies very quickly.
>
> Stephen Soloway, M.D.

After many denials for Remicade for another patient, and after speaking to several people, I was able to have a peer-to-peer on the phone with the insurance company. The "peer" got on the phone and said, "How did you come to the diagnosis?"

I said, "Well, this is a peer-to-peer and you are a rheumatologist. Just read my notes."

He told me he's more of an emergency room physician—in Ohio. He does that in addition to this job.

I said, "Well, okay. Then this is not a medical peer-to-peer. This is a financial peer-to-peer. In a financial peer-to-peer, there is nobody questioning my medical ability. I'm questioning your rationale because you are telling me I can't use Remicade. If I can't, I'm going to use Aria, which is double the price and given twice as much, so I'm going make many times as much money. I don't really understand. What doesn't make sense about that to you, since you are calling yourself a medical director? If you are not the guy fit for this, why don't you forward this to your company CEO or whoever's above you?"

"There is nobody above me in the department that would need to speak to you."

"I don't understand. It sounds like I appeal to nobody, which is you? Nothing personal, but you can't help me."

He says, "Well, I'm going by the guidelines." Ah, the guidelines!

I said, "The guidelines say the speed limit is sixty-five. Do you try to get to sixty-five in a blizzard? I'm just curious. How strict are you with these guidelines? Let me ask you something: You are an ER doc. A twenty-five-year-old girl comes into your ER with a submassive pulmonary embolus.

They're five minutes over the limit to get the clot buster. Are you going to give them the clot buster or not? Before you answer the question, because I already know your answer, my daughter went to the ER with a submassive PE three years ago, and she was five minutes over the limit in spite of me screaming through the phone, where I'm on staff at the hospital. They disregarded my orders and followed the guidelines. Now years later, my daughter still has this clot, for which one day she may need cardiothoracic surgery to remove it—because somebody was too stupid to think, and the person *followed the guidelines.*

"This is really what's sad about the guidelines. The guidelines are for people who are very dumb. People who can think write guidelines for the people who can't. You sound like a smart guy. You are on the phone having a peer-to-peer with a well-seasoned rheumatologist who has three times as many years of experience as you do—you 10, me 30. So I don't know where we are peers. We're not peers at all."

I was very polite to him! Of course, as soon as we hit thirty minutes on the clock he said, "I have to go. I have another appointment now."

I said, "What you mean to say is your guidelines are that you need to condemn everybody within thirty minutes."

He says, "Erica, who you spoke to yesterday for thirty-nine minutes, filed a complaint" on the company's complaint system.

I say, "So I spent thirty minutes plus preparation on a call today and another thirty-nine minutes on a call yesterday, plus five minutes wasted before and after. If I can see four people an hour; I've just lost eight people."

In the end, he told which two drugs their company allows, and he said, "I can't approve your drug."

I said, "Well, I'm not going to follow your orders. Not that it matters to you because you are in Ohio practicing emergency medicine, but what's going to happen next is I'm going to give out the home phone number and address of the CEO of the company."

"Oh, I wouldn't advise that," he said.

I said, "Sorry. It would be easier if you just approved the drug. But you are not. So what's going to happen now? I'm going to put the patient on Aria. I'm not going to use one of your two suggestions, and until my patient gets his correct drug, he and the rest of your people can't come here. I'm not going to treat them."

That's where we ended it. The guy thought I don't understand what's going on, but I'm smarter than he is. What's really going on is that most of the Remicade given in the country is given in the hospital. Anything administered in the hospital costs about 65 percent more than the cost to get the same thing in an office. They're not considering that I'm an office-based physician, not in a hospital.

The most charitable explanation is that the insurance companies probably believe they're denying these drugs in order to save money, when in fact it is going to end up costing more money, much more money. If they would simply listen to me and allow the drug to be given in my office—and stop arguing with me about the drug—they would save thousands of dollars per person—immediately.

I have been able to convince one of these insurance companies of this fact. In fact, Horizon New Jersey allowed me to switch 211 patients off of their preferred drug and back to my preferred drug.

But the situation is a classic case of stupidity and bureaucracy. This is an organization full of people who don't know what they're talking about and don't know when to listen to somebody who does.

Let us talk about guidelines. Hospitals, various physician organizations, other miscellaneous physician groups, and, most important, insurance companies often follow guidelines for treatment protocols. Guidelines are the most important way to limit the doctor's ability to think and are written by experts to outline the minimum knowledge required to tread water through a situation. The experienced physician would never follow guidelines. He or she would be capable of writing the guidelines and then using best judgment. But judgment is eliminated by the enforcement of guidelines. Sadly, some doctors must rely on guidelines. And with an increasing shortage of doctors, more and more doctors at triage-level positions can only follow guidelines. Many diseases have many different manifestations, which make the use of guidelines useless.

Here's an explanation of guidelines and their issues from Sean Weiss of Doctors Management:

Guidelines are just that: guidelines! They are also referred to as Sub Regulatory guidance. The difference between regulation and a guidance document? Guidance documents can't set "new" legal standards or impose "new" requirements. Unlike regulations, guidance documents don't contain amendments to the Code of Federal Regulations (CFR) and are not subject to the notice and comment process (typically sixty days). Guidance documents only clarify and affect how agencies administer regulations. It is important to keep in mind that they are not legally binding in the same way as rules issued through one of the rulemaking processes of the Administrative Procedure Act (APA).

Regarding guidelines, every one refers to what is "medically necessary" or "medical necessity," and it shall mean healthcare services that a physician, exercising prudent clinical judgment, would provide to a patient for the purpose of preventing, evaluating, diagnosing, or treating an illness, injury, disease or its symptoms, and that are: a) in accordance with generally accepted standards of medical practice; b) clinically appropriate, in terms of type, frequency, extent, site, and duration, and considered effective for the patient's illness, injury, or disease; and c) not primarily for the convenience of the patient, physician, or other healthcare provider, and not more costly than an alternative service or sequence of services at least as likely to produce equivalent therapeutic or diagnostic results as to the diagnosis or treatment of that patient's illness, injury, or disease. The definition of medical necessity in this case is that the term refers to "generally accepted standards of medical practice," based on credible scientific evidence published in peer-reviewed medical literature that is generally recognized by the relevant medical community or otherwise consistent with clinical consensus. According to CMS, "clinical judgement" is dependent upon two steps.

a. First, "The synthesis of all submitted medical record information (e.g., progress notes, diagnostic findings, medications, nursing notes, etc.) to create a longitudinal clinical picture of the patient."

b. Second, "The application of this clinical picture to the review criteria is to make a reviewer determination on whether the clinical requirements in the relevant policy have been met. MAC, CERT, RAC, and ZPIC/UPIC clinical review staff shall use clinical review judgment when making medical record review determination about a claim."

In further exploring Medicare's view of medical necessity, they establish a "legal doctrine by which evidence-based clinical standards are used to determine whether a treatment or procedure is reasonable, necessary and/or appropriate." In the Medicare program, "medical necessity" is defined under Title XVIII of the Social Security Act, Section 1862 (a) (1) (a): "Notwithstanding any other provision of this title, no payment may be made under part A or part B for any expenses incurred for items or services which, except for items and services described in a succeeding subparagraph, are not reasonable and necessary for the diagnosis or treatment of illness or injury or to improve the functioning of a malformed body member." The final aspect of medical necessity I wish to address comes from two cases with the first being heard in the Second Circuit Court of Appeals, as cited in Kaminski (http://www.cga.ct.gov/2007/rpt/2007-r-0055.htm), "Unless the contrary is specified, the term "medical necessity" must refer to what is medically necessary for a particular patient, and hence entails an individual assessment rather than a general determination of what works in the ordinary case."

*(Continued on next page)*

The second case is Holland v. Sullivan in which the court concluded, "Though the considerations bearing on the weight to be accorded a treating physician's opinion are not necessarily identical in the disability and Medicare context, we would expect the Secretary to place significant reliance on the informed opinion of a treating physician and either to apply the treating physician rule, with its component of "some extra weight" to be accorded that opinion, [even if contradicted by substantial evidence], or to supply a reasoned basis, in conformity with statutory purposes, for declining to do so." In further examining the "Treating Physician Rule" we look at the first section of the Medicare statute which is the prohibition, which states, "Nothing in this title shall be construed to authorize any Federal officer or employee to exercise any supervision or control over the practice of medicine or the manner in which medical services are provided." From this, one could conclude that the beneficiary's physician should decide what services are medically necessary for the beneficiary, and a substantial line of authority in the Social Security disability benefits area holds that the treating physician's opinion is entitled to special weight and is binding upon the Secretary when not contradicted by substantial evidence. Some courts have applied the rationale of the "treating physician" rule in Medicare cases, and have rejected the Secretary's assertion that the treating physician rule should not be applied to Medicare determinations. Defining medical necessity, "As program after program has evolved, there has developed a degree of complexity . . . regulations which make them almost unintelligible to the uninitiated . . . [a] draftsman who has gotten himself into a position requiring anything like [§139a(a)(10)(A)(ii)(VIII)(cc)] should make a fresh start." *Friedman v. Berger*, 547 F.2d 724, 727, n.7 (2d Cir. 1976), *cert. den.*, 430 U.S. 984 (1977). "[O]ne of the most completely impenetrable texts within human experience" and "dense reading of the most tortuous kind." *Rehab. Association of Virginia v. Kozlowski*, 42 F.3d 1444, 1450 (4th Cir. 1994).

It's beyond frustrating. My reputation is based on getting people better with the best product. Additionally, I accept the same amount of money for the regular drug as the generic. So there is no financial incentive for me to use one drug over another. This is pure corporate stupidity.

But who has time to write sixty letters? The key point is how much time I have to waste. It takes the same amount of time as six visits to see one patient in person and hassle to get that person treated properly. No amount of compensation would make this financially worthwhile. It's worthwhile because it's the right thing to do. The patients deserve the best care, and the insurance companies think they can harass people into accepting their injudicious decisions.

I'm not in medicine to save an insurance company money. Everybody thinks doctors should be worried about cost. I'm not worried about cost. I'm worried about the best treatments. You come to see me, you have insurance, I take it. We need to get you the best treatment. There is such extraordinary waste in the system. It is insane how the insurance companies think they are doctors and know what's best for patients without seeing them.

Isn't every person and diagnosis different? One patient of mine has GHI Insurance, a.k.a. EmblemHealth. The patients were denied coverage because the medication would exhaust the pharmacy benefits.

Another patient was denied medication and not covered because the insurance company said it was *not a medical necessity*, even though the *patient met all criteria* for the medication. The list of these denials goes on and on.

Here is another one. (I have hundreds!) A patient with dermatomyositis who met the typical criteria of proximal muscle weakness; typical rash, namely Gottron lesions; shawl sign; and creatine phosphokinase (CPK) of greater than 12,000 had been given a month of oral steroids and methotrexate with minimal change. IVIG was ordered to be given; however, it was denied by none other than Magellan Health, the pharmacy benefit manager for Blue Cross.

I called Magellan's 800 number and received a woman in Florida, who transferred me to a gentleman who identified himself as a pharmacist for

Magellan operating in Saint Louis. He advised he would be able to arrange for a peer-to-peer call for me. But after reading my note, he didn't see any problem, though he had no authority.

He admitted that the guidelines followed at both Magellan and Blue Cross are far behind the science and quite outdated; however, he still had to follow protocol. I explained that the patient's life could be in jeopardy, that I would be giving the drug regardless, that I would not hold the patient responsible. I merely stated I would file a lawsuit against the insurance company and report the company to the insurance commissioner. I would go after their credentials and their finances because they are disrupting the care of an innocent twenty-one-year-old man who has a rare disease, though it is not rare in my field and very treatable as long as it is treated on time and quickly.

This type of nonsense makes medicine difficult, and if you are asking why somebody didn't make the call for me, my staff does not understand medicine at the same level I do. The other request I had for the peer-to-peer is that I speak to a practicing rheumatologist, not the typical retired gynecologist or geriatrician or nursing home physician or part-time ER physician. I need somebody who might actually understand what I am talking about.

In response, I wrote the following letter to the president and CEO of Horizon Blue Cross Blue Shield of New Jersey:

TO: Gary D. St. Hilaire, President and CEO, HBCBSNJ

RE: Josue D.

Although ludicrous and redundant, here I am again. [Patient] has dermatomyositis, diagnosis made by proximal muscle weakness performed by a board-certified rheumatologist, CPK greater than 12,000 with no other cause, and anti-Mi-2 antibodies markedly elevated. This is the diagnosis of dermatomyositis, and for the past several decades a muscle biopsy is not required in this situation.

Sadly, I need to write and explain this. Why the health companies cannot keep up with the latest data or jargon is beyond my understanding. Why I have to waste time constantly to go above and beyond for my patients to give regular average standard normal care I don't know.

I will be giving this gentleman his IVIG as it is required, and I will not be getting or subjecting him to a biopsy which he does not need. He will be receiving his medicine with no authorization, and I do fully expect to be paid for that and for my inconvenience. You can add a 10% or 20% fee or we can go to court, or I can stop seeing your patients, or maybe there are other possibilities.

I do not understand why it is so difficult to do the right thing when there are so many people allegedly educated and intelligent that are involved. This is absolutely not the case, and I am tired of writing letters. They will look great in my book, but they will look badly upon your company.

I am not going to do a peer-to-peer on something that is so standard of care. This is insulting and embarrassing for a board-certified rheumatologist with four board certifications to get on the phone with anybody other than myself to talk about this topic.

Sincerely,
Stephen Soloway, M.D.

I had already been fighting with the company on another patient, about whom I wrote the following letter to a colleague asking him to join me in the fight:

TO: Jeffrey R. Boxman, D.O.
Dear Dr. Boxman:
I took your advice regarding [Patient]. I increased her IVIG to double dose; however, the insurance company denied the dosing. I want you to be

*(Continued on next page)*

aware I will be sending an FU letter to the insurance company. Please join me in attacking insurance companies as they have no precedent to deny your suggestion.

Sincerely,

Stephen Soloway, M.D.

The very same day I sent the letter to Dr. Boxman, I sent the following letter to Magellan:

TO: Magellan RX Management

RE: Denial of increased dose of IVIG

As you are aware, I am treating [Patient] for lupus and neurologic problems. At the request of her venerable neurologist, Dr. Boxman, doubling the dose of IVIG was recommended. However, there is a denial to the request. I bring this to your attention because I am certain it is an oversight. As you are aware there are no guidelines for lupus cerebritis, nor are there guidelines or indicated drugs for lupus cerebritis or immune neuropathy. We are not requesting the drug for her hypogammaglobulinemia. We are requesting it to treat her neuropathy related to lupus. So, unless you can come up with a better treatment plan for which we have exhausted all options, including the addition of cyclophosphamide which can be and will be combined in this patient, I insist that you overturn this error. Please note that I am an appointee of the President of the United States for health advice as well as the Chairman of the New Jersey State Board of Medical Examiner Preliminary Evaluation Committee, and the Chairman of Rheumatology at the Inspira Health Network.

Thank you kindly for your consideration,

Sincerely,

Stephen Soloway, M.D.

As if I hadn't spent enough time fighting for my patients that day, there was room for one more, this time about a denial for Rituximab:

TO: Magellan RX Management

The patient has confirmed aortitis. I have written to Omni Blue Cross and now I am filled with disgust. The patient is seen here today complaining of shortness of breath, fatigue, weakness, pain, and fever. He has known aortitis. He responds to steroids. He has been denied Rituximab. His working diagnosis is IgG4-related disease. It is impossible to biopsy the aorta, and even the most disingenuous of you reading this letter would understand that biopsy of the aorta is dangerous. In case you are not aware, the aorta is the largest blood vessel in the body and a biopsy would cause the patient to die. I attempted to get the patient Rituximab several months ago and provided articles, up-to-date articles in fact from rheumatology literature, but in spite of that the patient was denied.

The differential diagnoses for aortitis are small. It includes IgG4-related disease, retroperitoneal fibrosis, Behcet's disease or relapsing polychondritis with onset of aortitis, extracellular giant cell arteritis, and Erdheim Chester disease. Erdheim Chester disease is treated with Interferon; however, this disease has been excluded. Extracranial giant cell arteritis is treated with steroids and Tocilizumab; however, the patient is likely too young to have this. The patient has never exhibited the features of Behcet's disease or relapsing polychondritis, thus we cannot use these as a working diagnosis as it does not make sense. He does not have retroperitoneal fibrosis based on imaging; thus we are left with a working diagnosis of Ig4-related disease. With his new symptomatology and worsening symptomatology and now elevated hemoglobin and hematocrit, he will now need a hematology evaluation, although these may be elevated merely because he is short of breath. You are cutting off your nose to spite your face.

*(Continued on next page)*

Since there is nobody reading this letter and nobody within your company who would know more about this topic than myself, I would suggest that you put your bank account on the back burner and pay for this man's treatment.

I have already helped him obtain an attorney and I will back him as far as necessary. If I need to treat him against your guidelines, I will do that, and you will pay the bill. I assure you, you will pay the bill. I am very intelligent, calculated, and have extreme leverage. Please do not ever underestimate my ability when I am vigilant about a situation. In no uncertain terms you have angered me to a limit that I have not achieved in decades. Be forewarned, you will hear from me and the attorney again. Furthermore, should this not be resolved quickly I will have senators and congressmen camped out in front of your office and bring all major news outlets. If you are not aware, I am an appointee of the President, and the Chairman of the South Jersey PEC, a division of the Board of Medical Examiners. I am the Chairman of Rheumatology at Inspira Health Center, and many other accolades that are not worth my time to write here.

Please get the lead out and fix this man's ability to get proper care. Any injustice to him will place blood in your hands.

A month later, another letter on behalf of the previous patient:

[February 15, 2021, letter to Magellan re: Boxman/IVIG]

TO: Magellan Rx Management

Attn: Appeals Department

To Whom It May Concern:

I am sure you are doing well if you are reading this letter. Fortunately for you, you are doing better than [Patient]. While you are doing well, the level of intelligence and decision-making at Blue Cross is becoming frustrating. [Patient] has lupus with central nervous system involvement and dysautonomia, and at the advice of her neurologist Dr. Boxman he advised her IVIG being prescribed for hypogammaglobulinemia in the setting of her CNS lupus be doubled to 2 mg/kg. [Patient] had been clinically stable on 42 grams per month; however Blue Cross is only paying for 30 grams per month. This is not even the typical 1 mg/kg per day every two weeks, or what was formerly given as 400 mg/kg daily times five days. We are now prescribing it in a more effective and cost efficacious manner; however, as the primary care rheumatologist in this case I am deferring and agreeing with the neurologist who is suggesting her dose be doubled with scientific evidence to back up his claims, and you are punishing the patient.

This type of negligent behavior cannot be tolerated. I am certain that you will do right by [Patient] so she can feel as well as you do. I expect I will not have to take further action.

Thank you.


Stephen Soloway, M.D.


Five months later, I wrote another:


[June 1, 2021, letter to Magellan re: Rituximab]

TO: Magellan Rx Management

Attn: Appeals Department PO Box 1459

To Whom It May Concern:

With alarming concern Rituximab was denied by Blue Cross. This unprecedented unilateral decision does not fit with my practice. The patient is under my care, the patient is not under the care of the insurance company. If the insurance company has new policies, they must notify the

*(Continued on next page)*

physician in advance. The unilateral decisions will be overturned immediately, or they will be met with a nuclear triad of attacks. I will have
countless newspapers, medical boards, and attorneys all at your doorstep.
This is no joke. I take care of more Blue Cross patients in New Jersey than
anyone. Unless the CEO of the company or somebody who can act as a
surrogate sits with me in person, we would rather continue to give good
care or simply not see your patients again.

I wish you good luck finding anyone who provides the volume and
complexity of my practice. I realize quality is not an issue. Passing papers
and making money is the political issue here. That does not fly at this
office. You should be well advised, and you should be well versed with
who I am. I suggest you do your homework and call back with a favorable
response as the patient will not suffer, and if made to suffer will be forced
to go elsewhere.

Sincerely,
Stephen Soloway, M.D.

## United

The following letter was written to UnitedHealthcare after the company
refused to pay for reference medication. It would only allow for biosimilars.
I agreed to accept the price of the biosimilars even if I had to pay more to buy
the reference drug. I feel the reference drug is better and have no financial
motivation to use it. Yet the company always wants to exert whatever menial
power it can, which ultimately affects the care of their clients who pay the
premiums.

[December 28, 2020, Letter to UnitedHealthcare Oxford, Bhatnagar]

TO: UnitedHealthcare Oxford

ATTN: Upasana B., MD F.A.C.O.G., Chairperson, UnitedHealthcare Pharmacy & Therapeutics Committee

Dear Doctor:

I am the President and CEO of Arthritis and Rheumatology of South Jersey, one of the largest freestanding Rheumatology practices in the United States. I provide care for tens and thousands of patients including UnitedHealthcare patients. I am the Chairman of the South Jersey Preliminary Evaluation Committee, Board of Medical Examiners, New Jersey State Division of Consumer Affairs, Chairman of time Rheumatology Division at Inspira Health Network and Appointee of the President of the United States.

I *have* received your hostile letter which flabbergasted me. It is spiteful, nefarious and appalling. It is an egregious complicit assault to financially control my practice. I'm sorry to say, you *have* run into the wrong guy. I will be treating my patients correctly and I will not be adhering to your formulary. If this is not in concert with my office policy, then your patients will no longer be treated at my practice. I will transfer your patients to another insurer faster than a blink of an eye. If United Healthcare does not negotiate further steps to mitigate the proper practice of medicine, I will cease to do business with you immediately. I advise you to read my book titled *Bad Medicine: The Horrors of American Healthcare*, released about two months ago. I am an award-winning author, patent holder, inventor, and one of the top clinicians in the United States.

The state of New Jersey does not allow for transfer of biologic to biosimilar once the patient is already established on a TNF inhibitor. Here is an example: Remicade patients cannot be arbitrarily transferred to

*(Continued on next page)*

Infliximab generic. In fact, if that were the law, every company would mandate that; however, in New Jersey it is against the law. How do I know this? I am on the New Jersey State Division of Consumer Affairs. If I were to capriciously switch all my patients from one TNF inhibitor to another one, I would be audited and criminalized as doing this for financial gain.

Your letter states "Notice of Changes to Notification/Prior Authorization Requirements for Infliximab (Avsola, Inflectra®, Remicade®, and Renflexis®) Effective February 1, 2021." This unilateral decision is financially motivated at the cost of patient care. However, you have failed to mention you still have as first-line therapy other TNF inhibitors such as Simponi Aria® (Golimumab). If you would like to come to an agreement, rather than switching to drugs that I will not stock in the practice, I will NOT switch your patients to Golimumab which is on your formulary as a Tier 1 product and much more expensive.

Being aware that I would be audited and possibly criminalized for subjectively switching patients from one TNF inhibitor to another with no medical justification would make me technically a rule breaker.

Unfortunately, your company policy is making me be a rule breaker for your financial benefit. Your letter states I have to change patients who are stable with their course of treatment to drugs of your choice because you say so. This conduct cannot be tolerated, and no patient will be switched from their current drug if they are stable. Going forward, if you wish to negotiate what drugs patients can go on, we can review that on a case-by-case basis. However, not adhering to my medical expert decision making will result in immediate cancelation of your contract with my practice. You are doing a disservice to your community, your country, and anyone who possesses your insurance other than the board of directors and shareholders of your company.

Sincerely,
Stephen Soloway, M.D.

This is UnitedHealthcare's response:

[February 9, 2021, letter from UnitedHealthcare to Dr. Soloway re: Infliximab]

Dr. Stephen Soloway, MD, FACP

Re: Your inquiry about UnitedHealthcare's coverage policy for Infliximab products

Dear Dr. Soloway:

. . .

In your letter, dated December 28, 2020, you shared concerns regarding the commercial policy requirement to transition existing utilizers of Remicade to one of the preferred biosimilars, Avsola or Inflectra.

Renflexis remains non-preferred.

[Author's note: This is for their financial benefit. Why do they feel no one is entitled to make a living except them? And shouldn't patients with this crap insurance know that they are pawns?]

We appreciate your insights and want to give you some background information.

*Medical and drug policy development*

Clinicians with subject matter expertise help us develop our medical and drug policies, as do materials and insights we receive from clinical experts. We review each submission with great care and consideration because they contribute to the overall quality and integrity of our medical policy review and development process.

*Biosimilars*

Biosimilars create a more competitive pricing environment among drug manufacturers while maintaining treatment standards. We evaluate each innovator (original biologic) and its biosimilar one by one and make strategic management decisions based on the lowest-cost product. Sometimes

(Continued on next page)

that means preferring the biosimilar, and sometimes it means preferring the innovator biologic. These decisions can help lower costs for our clients and members to improve access and impact health outcomes.

*Our current drug policy*

We take the safety of our plan members very seriously and carefully weigh all the evidence before making any decisions. Based on the published evidence, our Pharmacy and Therapeutics Committee has determined the biosimilar Infliximab products to be therapeutically equivalent, defined as producing similar efficacy and adverse effects, to each other and Remicade for all current uses.

[Author's note: if that is true, why are not all biosimilars allowed with the same company?]

Existing prior authorizations for Remicade will remain effective through the end date provided with the authorization or until the date of the member's eligibility changes, whichever is soonest. Requests for a new prior authorization of Remicade after Feb. 1, 2021, will be considered on a case-by-case basis as part of the prior authorization process.

*State biosimilar substitution laws*

Many states have now passed biosimilar substitution laws that specify when and how a pharmacist may substitute an FDA-approved biosimilar for an innovator product at the time of dispensing. These laws do not restrict the ability of a health plan from preferring a biosimilar as part of a coverage review and benefit decision.

*We welcome your feedback*

We appreciate you taking the time to contact us and hope this information is helpful to you. If you have further questions, please contact us medical_policy_inquiries@uhc.com.

Sincerely,

Upasana B., MD

Chairperson, UnitedHealthcare Pharmacy & Therapeutics Committee

Here's my reply:

[Response to UnitedHealthcare]

TO: Upasana B., M.D. F.A.C.O.G.

[Author's Note: "F.A.C.O.G" means this doctor is a gynecologist, probably retired.]

Chairperson, UnitedHealthcare Pharmacy Therapeutics Committee

Dear Dr. B.:

I am the President and CEO of Arthritis and Rheumatology Associates of South Jersey, one of the largest free-standing rheumatology practices in the United States providing care for tens of thousands of patients, including UnitedHealthcare patients. I have received your hostile letter which not only left me flabbergasted, it is a backhanded egregious, nefarious, duplicitous attempt to financially control my practice. Well I am sorry to say you wrote it to the wrong guy. I will be treating my patients correctly and I will not be adhering to your formulary. If this does not follow your demands, then your patients will not be allowed to come here anymore.

Let me point out several things. The State of New Jersey does not allow for a transfer of biologic to biosimilar once the patient is already established on a TNF inhibitor. For example, Remicade patients cannot be arbitrarily transferred to Infliximab generic. In fact, if that were the law, every company would mandate it; however, it is against the law in New Jersey.

Second, if I were to switch all of my patients from one TNF inhibitor to another, I would be audited and criminalized as doing this for financial gain. Your letter states, "notice of changes to notification prior authorization requirement for Infliximab (Avsola, Inflectra, Remicade, and Renflexis effective February 1, 2021). You have made a unilateral decision that for your financial benefits, those are the only drugs that you will

(Continued on next page)

approve. However, you have failed to mention that you still have as first-line therapy other TNF inhibitors. As an example, Simponi Aria, also known as golimumab. So, if you want to come to an agreement, rather than switching to drugs I will not stock in the practice, I will be switching your patients to golimumab which is on your formulary as a tier one product.

For good measure, I sent a letter to the New Jersey Department of Banking and Insurance:

[February 17, 2021, letter to NJ department of Banking and Insurance re: Remicade and Renflexis]

TO: NJ Department of Banking and Insurance 20 W. State Street

RE: UnitedHealthcare Community Plan and Commercial Plan

Please see the enclosed letter from UnitedHealthcare Commercial Insurance Plan refusing to pay for a patient's medication, namely Remicade and/or biosimilar Renflexis. This is in spite of patients currently on those medications and stable. To my knowledge it is against the state law of New Jersey to force patients that are currently stable on medication to be switched to another medication. This unprecedented act of greed by UnitedHealthcare may lead me to drop their insurance. I bring this to your attention because without me they will not be providing access to care in southern New Jersey. I am the lone rheumatologist who still takes both their commercial and Medicaid patients.

Thank you for looking into this serious matter as soon as possible.

Sincerely,

Stephen Soloway, M.D.

My daughter has newly diagnosed type 1 diabetes. She wants a state-of-the-art insulin pump, which is FDA approved. Her insurance company, the same one I have problems with from a physician's standpoint, is prohibiting her from getting her device that is required for her active lifestyle. Why should it pay for the newish device if somebody needs it, especially if the FDA has approved the insulin pump in question? If you think this happens only to my daughter, can you imagine the regular person who does not have a father who knows who to call when and how to fight in the trenches and get things done? The regular patients—and there are only 300 million—have no chance at getting proper treatment. It occurs every moment of every day.

Here is the beautiful letter she wrote to her insurance company in response to its repeated and thoughtless denials:

---

Hello,

I am Alyxandra Soloway-Craner. I have done everything I am told. All I want is the insulin device I require. I can't worry what Express Scripts thinks or decides!

I will hire lawyers and go to congress and smear your company. I will go on local TV and have offers to do so. PLEASE, I only want my Omnipod without the headaches.


Sincerely,

Alyxandra

---

## The Insurance Audit and Preauthorization Scams

The insurance companies put in their contract that they are allowed to audit the doctor. This is acceptable to a degree. However, when the audit is for hundreds of charts rather than three or four charts, it becomes burdensome to the point where another staff member has to be hired. One would think if you were audited three years in a row under the same type of audit and the company found nothing wrong and everything to its satisfaction, continuing the audits wouldn't make much sense. Yet that's not the case.

I recently received a random audit for over one hundred charts from one of the insurance companies for no reason. It wanted them within ten days. Even with a staff of thirty, that would not be doable. Eventually, it will threaten to hold back money, and the audits will be coming faster than I see the patients. To tell you how disorganized the company is, it has even audited a physician assistant who has not been with my practice for several years.

Why is the company continuing to throw roadblocks? The answer is simple. It may pay, say, $1 million a year—a random number—to my practice, and if we exceed that amount, it may well decide that we are not allowed to surpass that number without being scrutinized.

Why can't it see the real truth? Its plans and tactics are so horrible that nobody, including the local hospital, wants to deal with it or take its patients. The company seems to make great profit, and its stock continues to rise as it collects money from all who are willing to pay. However, the participants cannot get proper care, and doctors cannot meet the standard of care.

I will cite an example: For decades, dating back to the 1960s, '70s, and '80s, the procedure of lumbar facet injections for osteoarthritis of the lumbar spine has been written about in a textbook *Low Back Pain* written by Borenstein and Wiesel (1995). They advocate for the use of lumbar facet blocks in back pain. Whereas lumbar facet blocks are often administered by pain-management physicians, I happen to be unique in that I was taught how to do them in my time at the VA Hospital in Philadelphia.

In fact, I have surpassed most in my thousands of facet blocks with tremendous success as documented by patients who have it done two or three times a year and always seem to get better. The insurance companies fight me on this. Some of the hurdles placed by the insurance company include forcing physical therapy upon patients, which is almost guaranteed to fail 100 percent of the time. Patients often cannot afford the copays so they will not go. If they do, they get worse and end up costing the system more money. Thus, the insurance company will prevent a $400 procedure done in the office and cost the system thousands. If done by pain management at the hospital or ambulatory care center, this same procedure can be several thousand dollars. Typically for such a simple procedure the patient gets unnecessarily anesthetized or given IV sedation—at $1,000. A facility fee is anywhere from $500 to $2,000; on top of all of that is the procedure fee, which is far more than I get. I simply get the procedure fee and nothing else. How I operate saves the insurance company an immense amount of money, although it prohibits this, because perhaps it is not used to a rheumatologist practicing in this area or, more likely, it simply doesn't know what a rheumatologist actually does.

Nonetheless, the patients are put in the middle, like children in a divorce. We tell the insurance company that since we are having prepayment audits, we will not see its patients. The company rep says, "You must see our patients; you have a contract."

We say, "You are not paying us; we're not seeing them." The rep says the company is allowed to audit us. We agree, but it is not allowed to not pay us.

It can, of course, opt to not work with me, which will only harm its patients because in some cases the patients have nowhere else to go. In all cases, the quality of care elsewhere is inferior. Regardless, it's the patient who suffers.

Preauthorizations and precertifications are destroying healthcare right now. If a patient comes into my office with pulmonary hypertension and I want to write for a drug, there are three classes of drugs, and they're very expensive. So even though the patient is short of breath and looking blue in front of me, even though he or she had an echocardiogram that estimates the PA pressure to be double what it should be, and even though the patient had CAT scans and MRIs, I'm not allowed to give the drug.

They have to get a right heart catheterization first. Of course, I can't find any doctor who's going to do a right heart catheterization because, to the doctor, it's a waste of time. I've actually had docs call me and say, "Stop sending me right heart caths. They're a pain in the ass for me to do, and I don't get paid enough to waste my time doing them."

Personally, I think they're very easy to do, but they are overregulated. When I was a medical resident, we would do swan ganz catheters, which is a catheter that would go through the vein into the heart and take measurements. Now it's practically illegal *not* to do them under ultrasound guidance. We never used ultrasound guidance and never had any complications. The ultrasound guidance is another step and another waste of money. They should, instead, simply train people properly.

You need a preauthorization for everything you want to do. I dropped one insurance company—the only one I've dumped—because it wanted me to get authorization to drain a knee, which is the cardinal procedure in my field. When a patient comes in with a hot knee and I drain it, I don't get paid because I didn't get a preauthorization. To my credit, the patients covered by that company still come to my office and just pay cash.

Here is a synopsis of everything that's going on.

A person comes to me, and they're sick: fever, joint pain, unknown illness, losing weight for a year. The patient has been to the family doctor, the ER, the infection doctor, and the oncologist, and, finally, the patient has all but given up. But someone has told them, "Please, try my doctor, try Dr. Soloway. He will get to the bottom of it."

I look through their history and see what's positive and what hasn't been done. I say, "You need this test because I think you have $x$." And I order the test.

Almost without exception, the insurance companies reject the test. Everything is denied. People will say, "Oh, you don't have anything to worry about me. I have the best insurance." But there is no insurance anymore: denied, denied, denied.

The patient is told the service is not medically necessary. I then get my staff on board. I get articles to prove that the service is medically necessary.

In one particular case, a girl came to me with what I suspected was Takayasu arteritis. I had to get the articles to document that the test I ordered is the correct way to find out. I'll send a letter that will say, "This is what the patient needs. Your feckless idiot, who doesn't know medicine, denied the test for no reason other than to save you money. You are denying the test and delaying their possibility of recovery. I'm ordering the proper test, but now I have to waste time, staff, and energy to find four out of four hundred representative articles." Usually the company overturns the denial.

I carbon copy Congressman Van Drew's health-care person on all the letters. I blind copy a couple of law firms, and I always put a threat in the letter. I say, "If anything were to happen to this patient, the blood is on your hands. I'll help them sue you. I'll own your company, and I'll fire you."

After they read my letter, I always win. I've never lost one yet. Occasionally, I've developed relationships with people at the insurance companies, but the biggest problem is that three to five years later, that person moves on.

My assistant, Denise, who has been with me for over twenty years, handles many of these fights. She had the following to say:

This year, I'll have worked with Dr. Soloway for twenty-one years. I work with him all day long. I assist him in the exam rooms with the patient. I enter all the information for the visit, what's called the HPI—"history of present illness"—and the recommendation, so the diagnosis, the charges, and any tests that Dr. Soloway orders.

I also do prior authorizations for medications. Even though the patient may have been on a medication for years, sometimes the insurance company likes to change what they're currently taking. Then we have to do a letter of appeal and prove this patient is doing well on the medication they are on.

Sometimes we will prescribe a medication for a patient and their insurance company or the pharmacy will send us a notification saying that the medication needs a prior authorization. We then submit all the information to the insurance company or to their pharmacy benefits. Then they'll come back and say it is not formulary. "The patient must try and fill x, y, and z first."

It's happening more now than it did before because there is such a broad range of biologic medications. I've seen this more in the last five to

(Continued on next page)

ten years. The insurance companies or pharmacies have contracts with the drug companies, and it's those drugs that go on the formulary.

Patients don't realize. A lot of them don't know why it's happening. They say, "My doctor prescribed this medication. Why can't I have it? He thinks that this is best for me."

We do all the fighting for them. The insurance companies deny testing for whatever reason they want. They just come up with excuses.

One patient came in for lumbar facet injections, which are not allowed without a hassle. I agreed to do them for free, since I was sick of it already. I called the insurance company and got a human that agreed to backdate an authorization. The patient drove three hours to see me. No one else thought outside—or inside—the box to assist him. Here's the letter the insurance company sent me:

Dear Dr. Soloway

Thank you for your patience. I've finished my review of the issue you brought to our attention regarding an assumption of the denial of a claim for services provided on May 5, 2022, for failure to obtain an authorization.

On behalf of Cigna, I sincerely apologize for the inconvenience and frustration you have experienced. I'd like to share with you the steps I took to investigate this matter.

- We received your letter dated May 9, 2022, on May 10, 2022.
- Authorization number A63801147 was requested on May 9, 2022, and approved on May 9, 2022. The authorization showed an effective date of May 19, 2022, as this is the requested date of service.
- The authorization has now been updated to be effective May 5, 2022, to cover the date of service included in the letter and as

verified by your office via telephone call on May 11, 2022. An updated letter was faxed to your office on May 11, 2022.

- We do not have a claim on file for this date of service as of today.

Simply unbelievable.

# CHAPTER 8
# WHAT MAKES A GOOD DOCTOR?

## Why Am I So Good and So Many Others Are So Bad?

People ask why some doctors are so good while others are so terrible. Well, how's it possible that if pizza is so great, it's not great everywhere? Why am I so good and so many others are so bad? I have my own technique. I know which needles to use and how to use them. I know more than most doctors and certainly more than most rheumatologists. All of that helps. But the real difference is that I care. It's a small thing, but it's everything. It feels so good to be able to help my patients, people who have been suffering for so long. It's the one thing that keeps me motivated through all the trash—that, and I want to be the best.

I asked one lady recently, "Why is it I'm the fourth rheumatologist you are seeing?"

"Well, I don't know," she said. "I didn't know you, and they sent me somewhere else."

My theory: I'm like Michael Jordan. The fans love me; the owners hate me. The patients love me. The other doctors can't stand me; they pretend I don't exist.

It is never for the benefit of the patient. That's the problem.

Take Fran C., for example.

Fran C. is the medical director of New Jersey Medicaid. I've known her a long time as a patient who has aches and pains and needs a knee injection here and there. Over the years, she has tried to help me with stopping some of the floods of audits and harassment from these agencies. She sees what I do, and she knows all about me. But she has access to everyone in the state.

So when her face started hurting, she went to an ear, nose, and throat doctor, who told her she was nuts. When her face really started burning, she went to neurology. They wasted another month and told her she's crazy. She felt like her face was on fire.

The day she came to me as a patient, I said, "You've got giant cell arteritis. You are going blind right now. You need to go right next door and get IV steroids, 1,000 milligrams—right now, tomorrow, and the next day."

The first thing you need is an index of suspicion. You must say to yourself, *It's got eighteen wheels, and it's carrying meat, so it's more likely to be a truck than a car.* When a patient comes in, the first thing you do is you look at him or her. This patient was in her sixties and white. She starts telling me her face hurts. So I asked her, "When did it start hurting?" "It started hurting X number of months ago." For argument's sake, it started three months ago. Immediately, I know that there was a change three months ago. Since it's above the neck, I start thinking the most common thing above the neck that's dangerous is giant cell arteritis. From here, I get to be like a sniper with the questions. "Does your tongue hurt when you chew?"

"Well, yes, now that you mention it, it does; it has been for the last month or two."

"Does your jaw hurt when you chew?"

"Yes. I have noticed that since this started."

"Are you losing your vision? Do you have an issue with your eyes?"

"You know, in the last ten days, I have been getting this clouded, blurry, weird glitch."

I said, "Okay, you have giant cell arteritis."

As soon as she was done with the steroids, she came back and said, "You know, I'm already starting to feel better." After three days her vision was normal, but she obviously still had eye problems. So she made an appointment, which took her two to three months to get at Wills Eye Hospital. The doctor said, "Yes, you have this. Yes, this guy Soloway saved your life and your vision. Tell him he's amazing because he did what others don't and can't do."

A year or two back, I got a call from a dentist saying she got my name from so and so. "I need you," she said. "I'll do anything if you can just help my dental assistant." I brought her in, evaluated her, tested, did this, did that. On the second or third visit, I came up with a diagnosis and started treating her. She went from disability to working every day.

I didn't hear much from her after that. Then not long ago I get another call from her. She said, "My mom is visiting from Egypt, and she's getting ready to go back. She's in so much agony. Her back is so bad that she's given up; she can't walk. She can't stand. She can't carry her luggage. She can't do anything. I'm desperate. Can you help me?"

Without hesitating, I said, "Yes, I can help."

She said, "Do you need to see the MRI? Do you need to see this? Do you need to see that?"

I said based on the story she told me, she's got arthritis of the lumbar spine causing stenosis. She'd described it classically. (By the way, if a person has to lean forward on the shopping cart, that's what is wrong, no exceptions. As soon as I heard those things, I already knew I could help her.)

She said, "I'm going to text you over the MRI." Her mother had been a patient at Penn, and on more than one occasion, she had had transforaminal nerve root blocks, which means people are not injecting in the middle of the spine, like an epidural. They inject the actual nerves that are leaving the spine. The MRI showed nerve root impingement on the right side of L4 and/or L5. On one occasion, they did a nerve root block of the one on L4, and then the other one on L5. The injections did absolutely nothing for her.

What was no surprise was that the MRI, unless you are reading with one eye open and one eye closed, showed how the arthritis in L4 or L5 was very severe. There was also some arthritis at L3. So I said, "Look, just please bring her here. Don't sign in, I don't want her money. I'm not charging her. Just bring her straight in; we're going to do an X-ray of her back so I can actually look at the X-ray. I'm going to put her up on the table, I'm going to give her the shots, and she's going to go home.

"What about putting her to sleep and all the stuff they did at Penn?" she said.

"That's just so they can make more money. You don't need to be put to sleep for these. I know because I've had them myself." In fact, I've let Denise, my assistant, do them on me while I'm awake, guiding her where to put the needle while I'm watching the screen.

So I put her mom on the table, and she was freaking out with anxiety. Then I did exactly what I said I would do. The daughter was in the room and watched everything I did. It took less than five minutes, including climbing on the table and getting off the table.

Three days later, I call the dentist. "How's your mom?"

"Oh, my God," she said. "I love you. I'll do anything for you. My mom is packing her suitcases. She's walking. She's carrying things. Her life is completely normal again. How the hell did you know she needed this?"

But this is the whole point: Things that are common to me, for some reason, are not in the algorithm. If something doesn't fall in the algorithm, people just don't know what to do. The old adage is, "If you are in Texas, and you hear hoofbeats, it's a horse." If you are eighty-five years old with back pain and you are having a hard time standing up, a brief exam and a few questions to make sure you are not paralyzed or have spinal cord injury is about all it should take. This is just as common as dirt.

Now, why do I know this and others don't? It's a function of the mixed training I received from two different teachers. One was very practical, and one was very scientific. But I would say that the skills were there from the get-go. My confidence rose, so that after I was in practice for about five or six years, I was almost as good as I am now. With five years of experience, you know you are right but you are not going to argue. When you have thirty years of experience, you can argue with anybody.

I taught myself how to do injections. Even my two program directors don't know how to, never did, and didn't teach me. I taught myself at the VA because I was inquisitive. I would bring the patients down to the X-ray unit, and I would just tell the staff, "Put the patient here and turn on the fluoroscope. I have to look where I'm going." The staff had no idea why I was there. It was the VA, and it didn't matter. Nobody paid for it, nobody cared, nobody asked. I went room to room and took all who had back pain down to fluoroscopy, gave them the injections, and they got better.

I once spoke to a rheumatologist in Washington, DC, a pompous asshole who is five or ten years older than me and wrote a textbook on back pain. I asked him once about fifteen years ago, "What do you think of lumbar facet injections?"

He said, "Oh, they work very well."

I said, "Really? You do them?

"Oh, no, I don't do them. I refer the patients to pain management."

"Why don't you do them?"

"Who's got time to do that?"

"Well, I do many, and I make a fortune doing it."

Not that I needed it, but I got confirmation from him that they work. I was curious. It's in his book as a thing to do. In fact, that was on the boards as a question. Somebody with a particular condition was described, and the answer was, "Do lumbar facet injections." Still, no one in my field does them. Pain management gets paid much more because they anesthetize unnecessarily. They bring in anesthesia and need an operating room. I'm saving the system thousands upon thousands of dollars per patient. Nobody believes what I'm doing. It starts an FBI investigation!

A lady came in not long ago, the last patient of the night. She was a fifty-two-year-old white female who looked to be in good shape, like she's a runner or plays soccer or volleyball. She looked much younger than her age. She said, "My knee has been killing me for two years."

I said, "Well, there is nothing like hopping on it and coming here two years ago!"

"My family doctor at the time sent me to orthopedics," she said.

"And let me guess: they operated."

"Yes. And I haven't been normal since." Go figure.

When Denise walked in the room, I said, "Denise, this lady had knee surgery two years ago because her knee popped or clicked, and they didn't do anything. But they operated to remove the arthritis, which you can't do. They told her they scraped out the arthritis."

That's one of the worst things you can do because it grows right back, the little spurs. You don't want to do that to an arthritic knee—you don't repair it unless the person's falling. But they went in, they did the surgery, and two years later—surprise—the lady is in my office with stiffness and pain, pain, pain. She also told me they were injecting something in her knee that cost $3,600 [likely platelet-rich plasma (PRP)—definitely not recommended!].

I said, "If I'm going to take care of you, you are not to go back there again. You are getting ripped off. You just said for two years you are in agony worse than you were before the surgery, now you are letting them inject some horseshit that the insurance doesn't cover. Don't go back there!"

"Okay."

I took a needle and said, "I have to inject your knee."

"Well, they just did it like a week ago."

"Did it work?"

"No."

I put my finger where they put the shot. "Look, let me put it in the right place, and let's see what happens." I put it in the right place.

She said, "When are you going to do the needle?"

"I'm done."

"That's not possible."

I showed her the needle. Denise was there. We were all, like, hey, he did it. She didn't feel it. I said, "Ma'am, are you starting to get the picture? You've been screwed big time."

She said, "Yes, maybe."

I said, "Let's check your other joints." I grabbed her wrist and then her elbow. I said, "Denise, listen to this." She had what's called tendon crepitus of the lining of the elbow, which was so thick and inflamed that you could feel it grinding as you move it.

"That elbow must hurt you."

"Yes, when you move it and you touch it, it hurts."

"Mine doesn't hurt when I move it," I said. "So that's a problem. Let me put some medicine in your elbow. You are not going to feel it, and you'll feel better." I did it, and she was better. I told her she had inflammatory arthritis. "Let's put you on some medication. Come back in ten to fourteen days, and we'll see how you are doing. But promise me, you are not going to go back to any orthopedic doctor."

"No problem. I promise. I'll be back here. I'll do whatever you say. I've been in agony for two years. Those two joints feel good now."

It's so common: she was told she had arthritis, and doctors told her they removed it. Even Denise was laughing because she knows: You are not supposed to scrape out osteophytes because they come back, as we know. You are not supposed to repair a meniscus in an osteoarthritic knee because it's been proven time and time again that unless the person is falling on the floor you don't do it. Neither procedure needed to take place.

I received a call from my friend of more than forty years. He had swelling and pain in one knee that was so bad he couldn't move or walk. He went to the doctor, and an X-ray was ordered. If the X-ray didn't show anything, he was told, he would need to get an MRI. The doctor told him to take Aleve.

You might say, "What's the problem here?" It's that nothing was done correctly. If somebody has traumatic pain and swelling of a joint, most likely it would be either an infection or crystal arthritis, which would require the rheumatologist to stick a needle in the knee, drain the fluid, analyze the fluid, and administer a medication. That, along with the person's other medical history, would help determine the most appropriate treatment. The X-ray should have been done by the rheumatologist, as he or she would look for chondrocalcinosis and not for a fracture, which is a long shot. An MRI is a total waste of money, yet it is ordered routinely and overordered for no good reason other than generating fake income in medicine.

The MRI is one of the more widely used techniques of wasting money. However, since doctors need to cover their asses, they order the fanciest tests even if not the most appropriate so they can keep the auditors and the government away. The government and the insurance companies incentivize this type of behavior, all of which wastes huge amounts of money.

This system is so backwards. It makes me sick to know that if somebody came to my office with the exact same symptoms, within seconds they'd have a needle in their knee. I'd be draining the fluid, having it analyzed, and giving a diagnosis immediately. Not handled properly, these situations will drag on for weeks or months, cost a great deal of money, and lead to unnecessary hospitalization and unnecessary arthroscopic procedures to drain what somebody thinks is an infection. A simple trip to the rheumatologist with the same-day appointment would solve the problem for pennies on the dollar.

Another patient was admitted to the emergency room with a painful swollen knee. Inappropriately, orthopedics was consulted, not rheumatology. Needle aspiration revealed a large amount of joint fluid. The patient was admitted to the hospital with a septic knee and was scheduled to go to the operating room. I received a phone call from a concerned medical resident who was curious as to my thoughts regarding such treatment, knowing I am a bone and joint specialist. I questioned him as to what the gram stain—a stain to look for bacteria on slides of fluid—showed.

"Doctor, the gram stain was negative."

I said, "Resident, how can there be a septic knee with a negative gram stain?"

"Doctor, I don't know."

"How old is the patient? Tell me something about the case."

"Well, Dr. Soloway, the patient is a sixty-five-year-old white female, severe pain, unable to walk for two to three days. Never happened before. She doesn't do gardening, and she had no other history to speak of."

I said she probably has pseudogout and probably needs a steroid injection to the knee. Most important, the synovial fluid needs to be looked at for crystals. Since orthopedics do not know anything about crystals, synovial fluid crystal analysis was probably not ordered. I said to check the X-rays.

More than likely, he will see chondrocalcinosis notated. The films were likely done lying down, and therefore any osteoarthritis would be underappreciated as the joint spaces open up without weight bearing, except for very severe disease. For one reason or another the operating room was cancelled or delayed for one day.

Fortunately, within forty-eight hours the patient started to have resolution, and the problem was self-limited. I communicated a clinical diagnosis of pseudogout to the resident; however, other crystals and a variety of diseases look the same. One diagnosis that seemed impossible was a septic knee. Septic knee is always the number-one consideration because it is the worst-case scenario. One should not have orthopedics seeing hot joints when it only knows of septic knee; the rheumatologist, though, can easily treat a septic knee without surgery and treat an aseptic knee with a steroid injection without hesitation virtually all the time.

Another patient had multiple years seeing doctors, with no diagnosis. She went to pain management and orthopedics three times each. I was the first rheumatologist she saw. Within five minutes of seeing her, I knew she had inflammatory arthritis. I treated her with Medrol. I confirmed sacroiliitis on further imaging, and six months later she was completely asymptomatic with TNF inhibitor.

Here's one more: the patient went for four years to a rheumatologist, to three orthopedic surgeons, a family doctor, urgent care, and an emergency room. On the first visit here, I immediately diagnosed the patient clinically with inflammatory arthritis. He came back 100 percent asymptomatic. He was also noted to have testosterone severe deficiency, and proteinuria, none of which was ever discovered previously.

## How Do You Know If a Doctor Is Good?

Imagine a doctor greets you with a handshake, knows your name, is aware of your history, and doesn't stare at the computer. Imagine the doctor takes an interest, asks many questions. Some may not make sense to you, but they make sense to an intelligent interrogator, which is really what a doctor is.

Generally, most doctors today suck. They don't listen to your history, are too busy typing data so the hospital doesn't fire them and don't know who you are. If you are lucky, you'll see a doctor as opposed to a student or his nurse practitioner. Then again, if you are not an intelligent patient, you'll think those people are nicer and forget that they're not as knowledgeable as your doctor. But if your doctor must stare at the computer, perhaps something there is what he or she calls "interesting"—which usually means the doctor doesn't know what's wrong.

Then you find yourself going to a specialist. Some of them are nice, some are mean, some are very smart, some are not. What matters to you is which specialist is the right one for you to see, the one who can find out the nature of your problem—what you call it and how you fix it and take care of it forever. If the doctor can't do that, it doesn't matter if he buys you a new car and throws you a birthday party; he's just useless. The good doctor needs very astute skills, both by asking questions based on the complaint and by examining to try to prove or disprove your thoughts. The doctor needs the knowledge of what testing should be ordered and of the analysis of these tests, whether blood testing or imaging of some sort. Imaging can include the analysis of body fluids, or it can simply be an X-ray or anywhere in between. If your doctor cannot perform these simple skills, that doctor is not the right one for you and maybe not right for anybody.

## The Future of Medicine

Thirty-five years ago, we learned a lot and had really good teachers. It didn't matter if we went to medical school at Harvard or in the Caribbean. We became well-rounded doctors who interacted with patients. We looked our patients in the eye, touched them, examined them, and helped with their anxiety. We could read their emotions. We could tell if they had sweat dripping from their palms.

In the last fifteen years, we have entered the age of the computerized doctor and the hospital model in which hospitals hire all the doctors and have them do triage work. As artificial intelligence and computer technology become more mainstream—provided that chips and materials are made in the United States—medicine in the United States may reach a point where the doctor becomes obsolete. The number of doctors required would be very minimal, perhaps only enough for research or other jobs, but not seeing patients.

Doctors are cost-ineffective for this new system, which, obviously, the government knows. As such, you will go to a kiosk, the kiosk will answer remotely, and a nurse or a clerk will assist with the answers. We see this now occurring in pharmacies and at all the urgent care centers popping up, both of which are dismantling the family doctor. The specialist such as the rheumatologist is being pushed aside by both the primary-care physician and the orthopedist. The fact that knowledge differentials don't matter seems to bother nobody.

What will medicine be like in ten, twenty, or fifty years? The gastroenterologist will be replaced by a robot that does the scopes and a computer that reads the results. The cardiologist will be replaced by a kiosk reading EKGs, and the technician doing the echocardiogram will merely wait for the machine to spit out the results. The nephrologist will be replaced by a more high-tech version of a dialysis machine with a combined interactive function.

We sit back and wonder why nobody is going into medicine anymore. Why are young, ambitious people going into tech or Wall Street jobs instead? It appears the writing is on the wall: the regulations are becoming so obstructive to the practice of medicine that patients are not getting the treatments they need. They are getting substitutes. Patients are not getting the testing they need, as it is a drag on the insurance company's bottom line. Neither the doctors nor the patients are happy in this dynamic.

I wonder if there are no doctors, who can argue about what medicines work better than others? Will everything—even cancer treatment—be fully related to gene therapy and automated treatment? Will all diabetics merely wave their hands in the machine, find out the number of their glucose, and have a jellybean move from a dispenser? Instructions will be spoken by the machine in thirty-nine languages.

The kiosk will take the complicated case and examine the blood, and a gene test will determine the problem, with a slip or pill generated. On the flip side, if the patient has something simple like a cold or high blood pressure, an algorithm and a nonphysician provider will act as a kiosk but eventually will be replaced, like a tollbooth collector has. Everything will be an algorithm and cookbook, with little need for the clinician-physician.

Although I'm not certain if these changes will have positive aspects, I believe that without personal interaction between a person who needs help and a person who can help, the quality of care will almost certainly worsen. It is no different than a relationship between a husband and wife, which requires more than just one night of making a baby. It requires staying together to build a family and growing forward and teaching by example, an experience robots and machines do not offer. No artificial intelligence will ever replace a well-seasoned clinician who has the skills to speak with patients, understand their feelings, and look in their eyes to determine what may be wrong.

The future is uncertain in medicine. Rising costs, lack of access for all including the wealthy, artificial intelligence, automated artists with computers that have been government-mandated to maintain records for government audit purposes are problems. Also, no evidence yet shows computers have made medical care better. This was a canard by the government. If anything, care has gotten worse, as doctors hurry through visits to meet the fifteen-minute time frame and get everything documented in the computer, whether it's relevant to the particular case or not.

Patients love seeing a doctor who will sit down and speak with them. Granted, not every doctor can spend an hour with every patient, and that is probably not realistic unless it is psychiatry. I feel bad for psychiatrists, who make $300 an hour while deserving $3,000 an hour. Good psychiatrists are worth their weight in gold, yet they are underappreciated and utilized incorrectly. They are being subverted by psychologists. Many psychiatrists will own or hire multiple psychologists to do the talking and listening, while the psychiatrists merely refill prescriptions.

No one knows what the future holds, only what the politicians seem to be planning. The experiment that's gone on over the past fifteen years has led to a disastrous outcome for patient satisfaction and treatment. The training of new young physicians is failing. If you are reading this book and have the unfortunate pleasure of being a patient—somebody who briskly runs in and out of your room with a computer does not get to know you, has no idea what's wrong with you, and basically checks with Google to find out what the prescription should be—you certainly agree.

Perhaps this seems to be the most cost-efficient way for the government to canard the general public into thinking that we do not have socialized healthcare. However, we do. Mark my words, as I see it daily: the private insurance companies are worse. They set stringent rules to what is not allowed to be done unless somebody is ready to die—and then maybe they can get a cookie if they follow the rules and do not die. As you've seen from many of my letters involving lawyers, CEOs, and government officials, fighting on behalf of patients never used to be necessary. However, now, to maintain the level of care of yesteryear, it is part of the practice, all while defending yourself from audits, investigations, and other trumped-up nonsense that has nothing to do with medicine.

Only the financial bottom line matters to the financial-industrial complex, which combines the White House, the statehouse, Main Street, and Wall Street.

Why do we follow rules? Who makes them? What makes guidelines important at all? What happened to experience, to bedside manner? Why do we listen to anything except our gut after we've all learned the same things from the book? We use our learning, which is a new language, to create our own skills from our own experiences. This will trump guidelines every time. Yet we allow insurance companies to dictate protocols, treatments, and medicine, all based on cost—not our clinical judgment as physicians.

## The Soloway Bills

We must do what we can do to fight the system now before it's way too late. To that end, I've introduced two bills, which I call the Soloway Bills.

When I was a patient in the hospital in 2018, I was given Narcan, which I should not have been given. (I wrote about this horrifying episode in my first book.) The Narcan order is written on every chart in the hospital—a so-called blanket order. That should not be allowed. Because of that blanket order, an inexperienced young nurse gave me Narcan because the bell went off, and my pulse was 40. However, sometimes my pulse is 38. The administration of Narcan has permanently altered my life. The first bill is aimed at preventing this from ever happening to someone else.

The second bill relates to the administration of saline to flush an IV, which should be flushed with heparin. Heparin is a blood thinner, but for this application the dose is very minimal, just enough to clear the clots off the tube. I can attest to that. If people flush tubes with heparin, fewer patients will get clots if they have indwelling IVs. I suffered a deep vein thrombosis (DVT) in my arm because I was getting saline. Now because the law hasn't been changed, I've announced that I am allergic to saline; I can only tolerate heparin.

When I was in medical school training, everybody had what's called a hep lock—everybody. One day, there was a shortage, and workers decided that the saline was a penny less. Because of that, people like me who have sensitive veins, people who have unknown clotting, get clots and all kinds of bad things happen to them.

Now, those against what I propose will say, "Heparin has a lot of side effects." For patients on IV heparin because they have a clot in the lung, the pulmonary embolus, then, yes, depending on the amount of heparin and the amount of time they are on it, there could be side effects. But the flushing of an IV with heparin every four hours? No one should get side effects.

I told two senators whom I contribute to that if I don't have this bill heard on the senate floor of New Jersey, they should not count on me for money in the future. I don't have a lot of money, but I have enough to leverage people that want my money! That's not a bad place to be.

# CHAPTER 9
# BEYOND MEDICINE

## World War III

We are now in World War III. World War III is very complex, dating back to FDR, Johnson, and most recently, Obama. The fight is happening on many fronts: Black Lives Matter, ANTIFA, social media, left-wing propaganda, George Soros, China, Russia, Venezuela, Cuba, Nicaragua, domestic terrorism, homegrown terrorism, imported terrorism, the funding of the police, gang violence, fentanyl and other illegal drugs, and border security, to name a few.

In 2020, China unleashed a virus. You don't make these things by accident, and you don't play with them by accident or because you want to find out what they do.

(It is not unreasonable to think China is behind monkeypox as well. The first case of monkeypox was in 1970, but the virus was discovered in the late 1950s. It sat in a lab for years. Now, suddenly, cases are rising.)

The government did not handle COVID correctly. You can blame Dr. Fauci. The way to stop the virus would have been to distribute hundreds of millions of units of military-grade protective gear to all US citizens. This was either too time-consuming or too expensive. Regardless, they should have had distribution centers giving every US citizen military-grade protective gear.

You don't see soldiers getting deployed with N95s. They don't work in biochemical warfare. Why weren't they distributed throughout the country when the hospital ships were coming? Apparently, the ships were less expensive than the military-grade masks!

The Chinese are cunning. The Wuhan virus lab was run by the United States. Why was it run in Wuhan? Because we don't want that shit over here! China's people are all disposables on my scale of disposables and inter-changeables. So they turn over the lab to China. China does some extra experiments. It has to test the virus, so it does so on the Hong Kong protest-ers to thin the crowd. It worked so well, that China thinned out the American money. Then it could fight a proxy war by funding Russia because Russia is broke.

China caused this pandemic and knows Biden is going to print $10 tril-lion. Now the United States is weak and just can't print any more money. Without that option, the United States can't stimulate its economy, which leads to a horrendous inflation crisis, which the country is on its way to.

The situation is not about US politics as much as it is about our country. The United States may not be the world superpower anymore. Even if Russia fights a proxy war for China, it's another way of trying to test US boundaries. China built up weaponry in the South China Sea. What did the United States do? It did nothing. Taiwan is a sitting duck. Our country needs to send Taiwan everything, including cluster bombs with nuclear warheads.

China has three million Muslims in concentration camps simply because they're Muslim. It locked up twenty-five million people in Shanghai in a "lockdown." If the people were armed, maybe that wouldn't have happened. China will end up being the most powerful, most authoritarian country of all time.

Why isn't the government preparing us now for the potential onslaught of an invasion from China? Why doesn't the United States have a cyber force instead of a space force? A cyber force would be a lot more important than the space force. I think CENTCOM can destroy incoming nuclear missiles from afar; however, the military is woefully unprepared for conventional conflict. Our country is outnumbered and rapidly falling second to the Chinese in most technologies. I am not a military strategist; however, if the Chinese have announced the future wars will be fought with bioterrorism, cyberterrorism, and laser weaponry, I hope I am part of the masses that do not know the United States still has an edge in those fields. I suspect the United States has some edge, as the Chinese have not waged war on Taiwan quite yet.

Let's discuss COVID-19 and war. The pandemic was handled poorly with respect to distancing and masking. It was handled very well with respect to vaccination. I believe poor medical care in the hospitals caused more deaths than were reasonable; however, doctors were working in uncharted waters and were overwhelmed and overloaded.

The reason half the people died at the beginning of the pandemic is that they were inappropriately treated and ventilated. After seven days, an endotracheal tube needs to come out either to be changed or replaced with tracheostomy. People went for six weeks on a ventilator. Of course, even if they were going to live, they couldn't because when people pull the tube out, they are pulling out patients' lungs. When I got sick, I was smart enough to stay home and just take my chances.

Measures are done in the name of taking away our freedom. The government tells us we have to wear masks. There is no scientific basis for doing that. In 2020 my office staff wore masks, gowns, and gloves. In spite of it, we all got COVID-19—and were quite sick.

Making people wear masks was a knee-jerk reaction that allowed the government to say it was doing something. The government is a good talker but not a good doer. The only masks that would have done anything are those given to the soldiers to protect against chemical and biological weapons. But the N95s were never going to do anything. This mask keeps out 95 percent of particles 3 μm or more; the virus on is 0.9 μm. Skeptics may argue the viron might be attached to a larger airborne particle.

One thing is clear: It is a dangerous world and it's only becoming more dangerous.

For the last eighty years, the medical profession has accepted the psychiatry bible, the *Diagnostic and Statistical Manual of Mental Disorders*, or DSM. The DSM-IV lists transgender as a mental illness, whereas the DSM-V does not. If this is not an example of rewriting the rules to fit a particular agenda, then there is no more reality. We allegedly live in a free nonbarbaric society in which any sector of the population is accepted and is protected by the constitution against harassment and such.

A case of a transgendered swimmer made news recently; whether this individual is a man, woman, or something else does not matter. What matters is the individual was born with an XY chromosome and was therefore born a male and chose to become a female. However, again woke society—the NCAA in this case—did not protect the cis women. This cannot be fair. Despite all the talk, the reality is that XY equals male, and XX equals female.

People of any sex, religion, and creed should be allowed to participate in any sport—however, only with their own kind. Men do not swim with women and women do not swim with men. In something as important as a nationally sanctioned event, people with male genitalia do not change in the female dressing room simply because they have said they are now women. It is shameful and embarrassing that the NCAA did not take a strong position here, but fortunately Fédération Internationale de Natation (FINA) did. FINA decided one must undergo hormone replacement therapy before the age of twelve to be allowed to participate as the opposite sex. I believe a segment of the Special Olympics should be made for all who question, or want to change, gender.

Regardless of what the DSM-IV or DSM-V says, transgenderism has to be a mental illness. It is in fact a delusion, which is defined as a false, unshakable belief. Delusions, along with illusions and hallucinations, are the three features of psychosis. These definitions have been accepted for centuries. Under the backdrop of a leftist-controlled government this all goes on as intended. It is simply wrong, and I am not transphobic. Readers who think I am probably don't understand my message.

The pitiful handling of the situation by the Ivy League should not be overlooked. For the sake of winning races, the university that allowed this to occur was looking for TV money and other endorsements rather than the integrity of purely female sports. In another country such as Saudi Arabia, the athlete in question would have been put to death. If this is not addressed across all sports immediately, there will be grave consequences, including females boxing and wrestling males and possibly dying. The same will occur in football, lacrosse, field hockey, ice hockey, and many other sports.

Why isn't the transgender athlete automatically in the Special Olympics? Male is male, female is female, and transgender is transgender whether male to female or female to male. There is no debate here. It is every person's right to choose their identity based on what they believe they are. However, a false belief is a delusion. Those who believe they are something other than what they were born as should compete with others with the same mindset. Everyone deserves the opportunity to compete. Everyone has rights that should be respected. My problem is when a particular group decides it needs a parade and extra rights that others do not have.

Reagan correctly stated at any point we were fifteen years away from losing our freedom. It seems that in the last fifteen years with the onset of Obama—Barry or Hussein, whichever suited his agenda as president—something I can't put my finger on has changed. I'm not saying I blame him, but I'm not saying I don't blame him either. It would appear to the outside observer that he was the first non-Judeo-Christian-believing president ever.

The past fifteen years have led up to where we are today, which is in complete and utter chaos. Everything is out of control. It's embarrassing to say you are a white man in this country. There is something wrong with it, apparently, in today's culture.

The universities are out of control. It's an embarrassment to go to an Ivy League school. Three hundred and sixty thousand Chinese Communists are in our higher education system—medical schools, colleges, universities, and so on. I asked a government official, "Why don't we kick them all out?" The answer was, "Well, they would start asking for donations from everybody." My response was, "Then why don't we set a deadline where we don't take any new ones?" Whether they end up staying in the country or not, they're always sending the information they gather here back home.

If you suggest anything about throwing them out of colleges, sending them back to China, repossessing their land, seizing their assets, whatever it is, then you are labeled a xenophobe, a misogynist, a weirdo, and an asshole. You are not allowed to suggest closing the border. We're supposed to take in 18,000 people a day, but we can't take a million Ukrainians? We should send one of those COVID-19 ships—the Floating Hospital—to Ukraine and put as many people as possible on it before the whole place is burned to rubble. We should allow the Ukrainians refuge here in the United States.

Everyone has an opinion, but I always seem to be right. We're not protecting Ukraine, sanctioning Russia, or sanctioning China. The sanctions are not enforceable. We're not going to protect Taiwan. The border will not be shut; more Democratic votes will cross. The United States is not deporting illegal felons. What kind of a country has no borders?

With the United States having rogue leadership in the oval office, I wonder if the skeletons in Joe or Hunter Biden's closet stifle proper actions, such as arming Ukraine. Ukraine (a new democracy with the zeal of the early days of the American revolution), with Zelensky taking a page from Churchill and George Washington, is the first line of defense for Western civilization.

Regardless of how compromised our government is, good always wins. The Nazis were defeated, and Putin and those of his ilk will be defeated. When losing is not an option and the cause is righteous, the underdog will prevail.

Contrary to customary belief, the United Nations (UN), a rogue organization, should cease to exist. The same goes for international security services. War has no rules; a war is a death fight. All is fair in war (even if I don't agree): torture, WMDs, fake-flag operations, false ceasefires. Laws and rules that can't be taken seriously or enforceable have no place in this world.

In addition to our compromised POTUS, we now have our own oligarchs who I believe are pushing their agenda of American Socialists, Communists, and Marxists. In my eyes, these are all the same. Our government used its power to break up the monopolies of AT&T and Philip Morris. However, the American oligarchs are labeled as such not only due to the hundreds of billions of dollars but because they echo the voice of our ever-increasing overreaching government. No administration seems willing to confront and dismantle the Google and Facebook monopolies, which have taken away free speech. Conservatives speak of change. I'd love to see a Republican administration, or a fiscally responsible Democrat (an oxymoron), break up the monopolies and return free speech as it is guaranteed in the constitution.

The loss of free speech will carry over into healthcare. Doctors will no longer make choices on how to treat patients. Your friendly insurance carrier will dictate to your doc what treatment plan needs to be adhered to.

We are always making wrong decisions: our so-called allies—Germany, India—flood our medical system, yet their governments flood our enemies (Russia) with money through the purchase of oil. I guess these are fake friends!

We are not in a cold war. We are in a bona fide war—a World War. As technology goes, this is a cyber, chemical, and biological war. And geopolitics only ever comes down to "What have you done for me lately?"

The war in Ukraine should be of no surprise to anybody. Tyrants with nuclear weapons or weapons of mass destruction often flex their muscle at the expense of innocent neighbors. Since the dropping of the atomic bomb on Japan, the United States not been involved in an intelligent war. In the Korean War, the United States conceded to the Chinese. In the Vietnam War, nothing was accomplished, but our country did not mind fighting because Vietnam was far from a superpower. In Afghanistan and Middle Eastern wars that the United States has become bogged down in, generally nonnuclear nations with little or no bona fide defense have been the foes.

We are watching the genocide of Ukraine, and we are not stepping in because our president is either compromised by the Russian president or we are simply scared that we do not have the manpower, the money, or the weapons systems necessary to stop the slaughtering of these people. This war will continue to escalate and there will be tens of millions dead unless something is done now.

Why does this have to do with medical politics? Continuous wars fit the left agenda, as they fuel defense contracts, munitions, the pentagon, and the VA. However, simmering conflicts with China and Russia are out of our league as we slowly recede as the world superpower. This all relates back to our foundering economy, which leads to insurance companies, starting with Medicare and Medicaid, to pay doctors less, forcing the more intelligent people in society to apply to graduate schools other than medical school. This weakens the pool of the brightest and most innovative, who have obviously gone into tech or financial careers.

Similar to our military and our country's defense, where we probably rely on 50,000 really smart people to defend 330 million, in medicine, where we may have one million doctors, fifty of them have a waiting list a year long. Quality of care is going downhill while technology is improving medical devices. However, the current situation of hospital-employed doctors is that of 15-minute time maximums and lack of proper care.

The doctors are all worried about their RVUs and are paid based on this formula. Working for a hospital, you must worry about RVUs. Then again, a colleague called me and stated he was owed $2 million based on his RVU bonus, but the hospital that employs him would not pay because he was already salaried more than the average doctor for his particular specialty. How outrageous is that? What motivation does this doctor have to continue working? Also, the hospitals are paid significantly for having medical residents who are actual physicians not yet knowledgeable or experienced enough to go out on their own. Yet nobody is teaching them properly.

Sadly, because I am working more than most, I am actually accused of fraud rather than commended for my work. Most of my patient population has already been to two or even three doctors within my field or within orthopedics only to come here and wait several hours for a visit. They are diagnosed, treated, and happy. They mention the wait time, and I try to explain the time wasted was at the three doctors they saw before me! Most of the patients seeing me are wasting large amounts of money throughout the system by seeing doctors not experienced, poorly trained, or less qualified for any number of reasons.

During those visits, X-rays and blood tests are either unexplained or poorly explained, which leads to wrong treatment and diagnosis. This may actually be one of the largest sources of wasted money within healthcare.

The setup to monitor doctors is very flawed. Barely educated people are looking for keywords and charts with no understanding.

The government protects the larger institutions both on the state and federal levels. I filed a complaint against an Ivy League institution for blatant misrepresentation. The government hopped on it right away since I am a member of the federation of state medical boards. However, the ruling was that the institution did nothing wrong, and I was not allowed to know any of the details. Clearly, there was a cover-up. These large institutions that get government funding do not comply with the same laws a doctor's office adheres to. The private-practice doctor creates a threat to the government because he or she is a self-employed individual not dependent on somebody else—least of all the state. The left does not want people to be independent.

As the government continues to grow, more peasants will be just above the welfare or poverty line. These will become institutionalized or entrenched in what is leading to outright Socialism or Communism or Marxism, and they will be snitching on their neighbors (and their doctor) for any minor infraction that will get them an extra cookie in the food line.

As the situation deteriorates, what happens when crime goes up in liberal cities? The population of people who would normally go to a doctor leaves.

When they leave, the doctors working in that city lose business, and then they leave. The poor people are then left behind without health-care services. This becomes a vicious circle, as money shifts to the suburbs—the doctors and their patients both live there.

To make the system really work, financial security must be in the medical system, in the rich and the poor neighborhoods at all times, regardless of what the demographics are at any point.

When COVID-19 hit New York City, a million people left. They may never come back. Some of those people were doctors. What if those people that left New York go back in five years only to find out the infrastructure is gone? You have to keep the population, locals, and government officials on high alert, and the only way to do that is to have Medicaid and Medicare pay doctors enough to stay put and not bail out of taking care of people they don't want to take care of. They became doctors for the love of medicine, not money, allegedly. If you do a good job at something, you'll make money. If you have a passion for what you are doing, you'll do it well.

History and precedent are being destroyed in medicine. This is in line with the change in language with written and spoken modes of communication and ownership of media by oligarchs. HIPAA is destructive and creates fear, controversy, and animosity among doctors trying to communicate about a patient while a nefarious spouse can always find a way to get material from medical records.

The *New England Journal of Medicine* is a left-wing rag. Transgender people represent one 1,000,000th of the population. Why are they on the cover of this publication?

I saw an article recently in the journal called "Interviewed While Black." This is a medical journal! It is a disgraceful joke of a journal. Two-thirds of it are wasted on propaganda.

Look at the correspondence section of a recent issue, for example: "Racial bias in pulse oximetry measurements." Well, why is there bias? Is the machinery broken? How can there be bias? It's a test. How about just saying doctors expect different outcomes from different ethnic groups?

In the last ten years, this has become all the journals talk about.

The problem with this is that the attention doesn't go to the people that need the care. The attention is focused on the squeaky wheel. The left-wing MO says, "No, everything has to go to us. What do you mean, you are not writing about us? Nobody's going to know what to do with us." All the people with cancer who are dying and all those with untreatable mental illness leading to serial killings and mass murders (and people blame the gun manufacturers!) don't get enough attention. You have to forget about them and worry about the transgender people.

In twenty-five years of practicing medicine, I've seen one transgender patient. He came from New York, and the only reason I knew he was a man was because he was part of the accounting firm that serviced my practice. When he became a woman, he came back and said, "You know, you always seemed like a very kind, sympathetic man."

I said, "I am."

"That's why I'm here," he said. "Everyone else wants to kill me."

I said, "I don't want to kill you. I want to treat you! But I don't give a shit if you are a man or a woman."

Then he'd get angry when I'd call them Eddie instead of Emily. This is what the left wants, and medicine, along with everything else in our society, will suffer for it.

# CHAPTER 10
# RHEUMATOLOGY FOR DUMMIES

In my first book, *Bad Medicine*, I included the chapter "Rheumatology for Dummies." Because the waiting list to see me can be long and intimidating and not everyone can come to New Jersey, I felt it was crucial to lay out the answers to some of the most common questions I get. I've built a substantial following on YouTube, where I post informational videos and full lectures. I do my best to answer questions in the comments—questions that come from all over the world, from people who are suffering and cannot find a doctor competent enough to take care of them, and even from doctors in training. My YouTube channel can be found at https://YouTube/StephenSolowayMD.com.

In *Bad Medicine*, I covered rheumatoid arthritis and psoriatic arthritis to autoimmune disorders, gout, and lupus. These are all common in my practice. Here, though, I'd like to discuss osteoporosis, fibromyalgia, scleroderma, myositis, vasculitis, and other diseases that affect millions of people. In this and the following chapter ("Orthopedics for Dummies"), I will answer common questions—basic and advanced—and I will explain in detail why most people who end up seeing an orthopedic doctor should see a rheumatologist instead. So much time, money, pain, and waste could be saved if people understand that.

People don't know, and most doctors don't either. And the ones who do know aren't saying. In a broken system, an informed patient is a powerful patient. Patients *must* educate themselves so that they can advocate for themselves. If they don't, they will be treated like the interchangeables and disposables. That is, like peasants.

Here we go with rheumatology for dummies. I will explain where your pain originates from, why your muscles do not work well, and why you are at a high risk of breaking a bone. I'm going to discuss osteoporosis and explain why you don't have fibromyalgia. I will touch upon scleroderma, Sjogren syndrome, myositis, and vasculitis, all of which are common in a rheumatology practice. These are diseases that affect people in profound ways and yet are misdiagnosed, left untreated, or treated improperly all the time. The incompetence is ubiquitous. I *always* say that the rheumatologist is the most important doctor you can have. I'll explain why.

Osteoporosis is a systemic disease manifest by thinning of bone and increasing fracture risk. In the medical world, it is a bone disease. But what I tell patients—and what people need to know—is that the way to prevent bone loss is to maximize your calcium and vitamin D *before* you are thirty-five years old. This is "primary prevention" because a person's bone mass is completed by then.

Until you are thirty-five years old, you are building your own bone. If you are forty or sixty or eighty years old and you are taking a ton of calcium and vitamin D, you are more likely to experience side effects, but you certainly are not going to add bone. Calcium and vitamin D build bone in a healthy individual up until the age of thirty-five. Once you hit thirty-five, it's only a matter of time before your bone density falls below an arbitrary line called the "fracture threshold."

From age thirty-five to fifty, you maintain your bone. At age fifty-one (the average age for menopause), you have about a two-year window when you are going to lose about 80 percent of what you are going to lose for the rest of your life due to the loss of estrogen. (Keep in mind that most data is based on the postmenopausal female population.)

If your bone density is very high, you may not cross that fracture threshold until you are 120 years old. But, unfortunately, most people are going to get to that fracture threshold somewhere after the age of seventy-five. It varies from person to person. By and large, all people, once they are old enough, will fall below the fracture threshold.

We should be telling young people that they must take calcium and vitamin D now—*when they are young*—so they don't have to worry when they are older. But in reality, people who come to me past fifty often need to build bone because they're at risk of fracture.

If you wait until you are eighty years old, you miss the boat. Nothing is more annoying than seeing a nursing home filled and residents on oral bisphosphonates, which they can't tolerate. It's too little, too late. (Frankly, nursing home patients with almost no exception should never be prescribed oral bisphosphonates due to atrophic gastritis, the ubiquitous use of proton pump inhibitors, and their inability to cooperate and stand for thirty minutes to sixty minutes with no tea, coffee, toothpaste, or mint gum.)

People over fifty must take calcium and vitamin D too. If you are over fifty, you take calcium citrate, rather than calcium carbonate, because the older stomach has a better time absorbing the calcium citrate, even though the calcium carbonate—Tums—is more common, easier to get, and contains a higher amount of elemental calcium. Forego the higher amount of elemental calcium for the one that's easily absorbable in an elderly stomach. People need vitamin D to assist in the absorption of calcium and because it forms the subfloor of new bone, referred to as the osteoid seam.

Let's talk about bone physiology. Think of your healthy bone as a blacktop highway. It's snowing, and the plow comes in and it takes a chunk out of the highway. Where that chunk was taken out a new chunk is placed back in. In bone, that phenomenon is referred to as "coupling"; it's the remodeling of bone. Like when you get a haircut and your hair grows back, or when you cut your nails and your nails grow back, your bone is always growing. (When somebody has arthritis, the bones grow in crazy directions and they are no longer in the normal position; they're too close together, and the remodeling forms spurs, which are new bone growth.) With age, coupling becomes uncoupled, which leads to bone loss—or, more accurately, loss of bone density. (The osteoclast outperforms the osteoblast as we age.)

Building new bone *is not* the same as preventing fractures. We know this from sodium fluoride, the fluoride in toothpaste. When it came out in a medicine called slo-flo, it made massive amounts of new bone. However, the bone was fragile, and it *increased* the risk of fractures. Bone is hydroxyapatite, not hydroxyfluoride. The goal is to form hydroxyapatite for healthy bone. In general, you take your calcium and your vitamin D because you need them to support your healthy bone, not to grow new bone. But without the calcium and vitamin D, your body is going to steal from the healthy bone that you have.

Beyond calcium and Vitamin D, two classes of bone medications exist: prevention of loss and bone builders. The former are called bisphosphonates—Fosamax or Alendronate or Reclast. They inhibit the osteoclast. Think of that highway again with the chunk missing. The removing of bone is resorption, or the osteoclast function. This is normal. To refill the pothole, you first have to lay a sub-floor, which is the osteoid seam, or vitamin D. Then on top of the sub-floor comes the osteoblast. It lays new bone, which is the normal coupling process. Aging leads to uncoupling, which leads to low bone-density and increased fracture risk.

The guidelines—set, of course, by Big Pharma, by incorrigible insurance companies, and so on—say that to maintain the bone density, or to hopefully increase it, you need to inhibit the osteoclast so that less bone comes out and the same amount goes back in. That's how prevention and bone resorption drugs work. This will enhance the existing trabecular bone.

Bone builders or osteoblast stimulators create new bone. If you have really fragile bone (as with thin, elderly people on steroids and who smoke), or you broke a bone (severe osteoporosis), you must build new bone first. You have to start your treatment with a bone builder. If you have fragile bone, but no fracture, you can start with an osteoclast inhibitor.

Osteoporosis is characterized by low bone density with or without fracture. It is never correctly notated to be mild, moderate, or severe unless there is an associated fracture, in which case, by definition, it is severe. But you are only as good as your weakest bone.

For the purpose of diagnosis, a dual-energy X-ray absorptiometry (DXA) is performed. This will measure the bone mineral density of the hip, spine, and wrist. These areas have trabecular bone, not cortical bone as in the arms and legs. Cortical bone is long and hard, like a baseball bat. Trabecular bone is thin and spongy, like a mattress. (In fact, it looks like the inside of a mattress.) You can think of those pieces of bone-like struts between a floor and ceiling. When these struts become thin, fractures seem to occur for almost no reason. But it's because the network of bone density of the trabecular bone has become too thin. By using drugs like Prolia, a monoclonal antibody that binds RANKL, thereby inhibiting the osteoclast, Reclast, or Fosamax, you can enhance the existing bone. The other drugs, the osteoblasts stimulators, will actually create new bone.

If somebody has a DXA scan and a low T-score, which compares the individual to the thirty-five-year-old-female with normal bone—the young healthy female—the bone mineral density is $X$ number of standard deviations below the mean. The definition in the literature indicates a T-score of -2.5 below the mean or less is osteoporosis. The areas tested are the lumbar spine and the nondominant hip. The nondominant forearm is used in hyperparathyroidism, and as in the case for those with bilateral hip replacement, we like a second site, unless the hip is conclusively abnormal. Areas of importance are the femoral neck, total hip, 1/3 forearm, > 2 contiguous vertebra with similar findings.

For a thirty-five-year-old healthy female, for example, a T-score of -1.1 to -2.4 is called osteopenia, and -2.5 and worse is all called low bone mass. You only use the word *severe* if there is a fracture. If you have a vertebral fracture, or if you have an atraumatic wrist fracture, even if the bone density were normal or osteopenic, that person would be an osteoporotic because the fracture overrides the machine finding. The definition of osteoporotic fracture would include a fall from the height of one's feet which results in a broken bone.

False negative results occur due to increased bone growth related to osteoarthritis and calcified aortic disease as DXA cannot differentiate those from lumbar bone mineral density. When the machine scans the spine, various factors may alter the accuracy of testing. The DXA may not detect brittle bones. Therefore, an actual fracture will supersede the density on the scan.

These are the guidelines. There is also the reality.

Most data about osteoporosis originates from postmenopausal women. This is the largest group of at-risk patients that will end up requiring treatment, thus costing money, which makes a trial viable to a drug maker.

Although postmenopausal women are the at-risk group to be checked, all men over sixty-five and all those with risk factors are checked. (Risk factors seem to vary by insurance; different insurance plans allow a variety of different risk factors. If the insurance plan sucks, risk factors may not be relevant.) Some risks include smoking, alcohol, aromatase inhibitors, proton pump inhibitors such as Prilosec or Nexium, celiac disease, rheumatoid arthritis, adrenal corticosteroid usage, and hyperthyroid, Cushing's syndrome, mastocytosis, hyperparathyroidism. Thin Asians or Caucasians are higher risk. Family history and fracture history (with minimal or no trauma; being hit by a bus or falling from a building don't count) need to be considered.

The best treatment is primary prevention. Build bones as a young person with calcium and vitamin D. Drink your milk! Continuous adequate levels of calcium, vitamin D, and weight-bearing exercise may slow the further loss and assist therapeutic measures. Low vitamin D can lead to osteomalacia, which is treated differently from osteoporosis yet can't be distinguished by DXA.

I screen *everybody* with risk factors, not only postmenopausal women. I screen men over sixty-five too. They're known to get what's called senile osteoporosis.

For those who don't believe that men get osteoporosis, they absolutely do. My office screens men over sixty-five. The average sixty-five-year-old man comes to see me and he's been to fifty doctors for fifty problems. He's never been tested. It's the same thing with women. Unless they have a really zealous gynecologist who is screening for osteoporosis, most women have never been tested. As with everything else—it's terrible for the patient!

If osteoporosis is present, start on calcium and vitamin D. We often find that most people are vitamin D insufficient or deficient. Before treating osteoporosis, we have to correct the vitamin D deficiency.

The Z-score compares the person to the age-match control. If you are a person under fifty, give or take, we need to use the Z-score. If you are a post-menopausal woman, say sixty-five, with a T-score of -2.5, we know you have osteoporosis. However, if your Z-score is also -2.0, -2.2, or -2.6, we know you are losing more bone than you are expected to lose for your age. We have to ask questions. Are you an alcoholic? Do you have thyroid disease? Do you have parathyroid disease? Do you have celiac disease? Do you have mastocytosis? Do you have another disease that's causing you to lose excessive bone disproportionate to age-related bone loss? It is imperative to know if there is another cause for bone loss other than aging. Treatment often would be delayed if a secondary problem is discovered.

For example, a man has osteoporosis and you find out his testosterone is drastically low. His testosterone could be low because of aging or treatment of prostate cancer. If due to aging, you'll tell the guy, "You are tired and impotent because of your low testosterone; it should be raised, however medication will be prescribed to treat osteoporosis." A patient with prostate cancer who had hormonal therapy to lower testosterone on purpose cannot raise his testosterone. This will stimulate his prostate cancer.

Osteoporosis has no symptoms, just like high blood pressure has none. However, risk factors are involved. Probably half the people we test have osteoporosis or osteopenia. It's staggering how often this goes undiagnosed.

The guidelines, which are really for the novice, tell you what drug you can and can't prescribe. These guidelines are about price manipulation not about patient outcome. I like using the injectable drugs, because the oral drugs are impossible for a person to take correctly. The package insert states that a person taking the oral bisphosphonate, the most widely prescribed medications for osteoporosis, must not lay down for a minimum of thirty minutes because if it stays in the esophagus, acid reflux is going to destroy the pill there. The pill has to get into the stomach. The patient cannot brush their teeth (toothpaste will render the drug ineffective), drink tea, coffee, or use mouthwash. The patient can't do much, other than stand with an empty mouth and stomach. Otherwise the drug is not absorbed. The drug is like a magnet—virtually everything will bind it, rendering it disabled. A thyroid patient who needs to take Synthroid in the morning on an empty stomach can't take oral bisphosphonates.

The only way to get proper compliance outside of a lab situation is to use injectable drugs. People bed-bound in group homes come to me, and every one of them is taking an oral bisphosphonate. None of them are taking it upright for half an hour. You could argue that they shouldn't even be treated at all without injectable medication.

Why did no one tell you to take calcium and vitamin D before you were thirty-five? Bad medicine. That's where a three-dimensional rheumatologist comes in. A push for primary-care rheumatology happened twenty years ago; your family doctor would have been a rheumatologist who could help with any rheumatic disease. That ended up dying on the vine. I remind everybody about calcium and vitamin D and DXA!

## You Do Not Have Fibromyalgia! (But You May Have Dysautonomia)

If an individual presents to a doctor's office indicating they have pain throughout their entire body, they suffer from poor sleep, depression, anxiety, agitation, brain fog, altered mood, excess sweating, perhaps dry mouth, lightheadedness or passing out, then they are labeled as crazy or diagnosed with fibromyalgia. Fibromyalgia is defined as a pain syndrome and remains a diagnosis of exclusion of inflammatory pain and requires distinct trigger points without pain in distinct placebo control points. They are treated for fibromyalgia with medications indicated by the FDA for fibromyalgia, yet they do not get better. If a person does not get better it is either the wrong diagnosis or the wrong treatment. Fibromyalgia is a quick and easy label for the doctor that does not have the time or knowledge to dive deep into the patient's history. Individuals with pain on palpation or squeezing of placebo control points have what is called pain amplification. These patients are a little loopy, but they really do have pain, or they perceive pain. They would be treated by either a pain-management doctor or a neurologist who specializes in use of low-dose Naltrexone, or whatever the best treatment is.

Fibromyalgia is actually rare. Dysautonomia is common. And chronic regional pain does exist, but it isn't fibromyalgia.

In my experience—which is vast enough to be accurate—and in collaboration with Dr. Nicholas DePace, a renowned professor of neurocardiology specializing in dysautonomia, we estimate 25 percent of random office visits are undiagnosed dysautonomia and 90 percent of those diagnosed with fibromyalgia across the board have dysautonomia. While the cause of dysautonomia is not always obvious, it is highly associated with EDS or Ehlers-Danlos syndrome.

Dysautonomia is of enormous importance especially since it is either misdiagnosed or not diagnosed very often.

The brain is the central nervous system; the hands and feet are the peripheral nervous system. The brain tells the hands, "Pick up the pen, and write something." Then there is the autonomic nervous system, which I refer to as the "automatic" nervous system. Sweating, goosebumps, anxiety, flushing, random tingling in the hands or feet, color changes in the hands or feet, both mental and skin irritability, palpitations, fainting, labile blood pressure, breathing rate, pulse—all of this is controlled by the autonomic nervous system.

Someone who constantly faints might have postural orthostatic tachycardia syndrome, or POTS. A patient stands up from a sitting position and the blood pressure doesn't rise appropriately. The person gets lightheaded or passes out. Because blood pressure doesn't rise fast enough, the heart beats much faster to try to keep up before fainting. The volume of blood lies in the legs instead of coming up with you. That's a malfunction of the autonomic nervous system. We encourage all such patients to wear support garments to maintain the pressure, hydrate with water, and typically use alpha adrenergic medications such as midodrine and an anticholinergic nortriptyline. These medications address the most common reasons for symptomatic dysautonomia, namely sympathetic withdrawal and parasympathetic excess. One can think of the sympathetic nervous system as the gas pedal of a car while the parasympathetic nervous system is the brake of the car. Patients with dysautonomia seem to have pain all over and mimic fibromyalgia. The reason is twofold. Many of the patients have EDS or a hypermobility disorder which leads to early osteoarthritis and joint pain. The small nerves, which are inflamed or irritated—known as small fiber neuropathy—will cause the sensation of burning, tingling, numbness, and unusual sensations throughout the entire body. This can only be diagnosed by a skin biopsy and measurement of a small fiber nerve or sudomotor (sweat gland testing) which is innervated by small fiber nerves. These tests for confirmation are not easily obtainable, nor are they reliable.

These disorders are most commonly from sympathetic withdrawal, which means that the sympathetic decrease and concurrent parasympathetic excess.

Many patients have said, "I have Raynaud. Look, my hands are purple." (Raynaud syndrome, by definition, is five to sixty minutes of a reversible spasm of the artery going into the hand, the nose, the ear, and any number of other places. If you halt circulation to the finger, initially it blanches and appears white. After a brief time the oxygen leaves and the area, now purple, flushes when blood returns and looks red. This is called a triple-phase color response. If that happens from five minutes to an hour, that's more likely to be Raynaud syndrome, which can be benign or associated with connective tissue diseases such as scleroderma or myositis.) Most of these people do not have Raynaud syndrome, just like most people who think they have fibromyalgia don't.

The body is sealed together with glue, called collagen. So "weak glue"—meaning a collagen defect—can lead to all sorts of issues. If the eyes are stretchy, the patient is nearsighted. If the skin is stretchy, cigarette-paper scars may occur. If the blood vessels are stretchy, easy bruising can result. If the muscles are stretchy, a hernia may be more likely. If the colon is stretchy, diverticulitis is more frequent. If the lungs are stretchy, pneumothorax is common. If the spinal cord is stretchy, a spinal cord leak could happen. (Don't do an epidural on that person!) If the ligaments are stretchy there is an increased risk of sprained ankles, knee pain from the kneecap sliding from side to side, snapping and clicking of the hips and shoulders, dislocation of the shoulders, scoliosis, or spondylolisthesis. Why? At birth, the bone that was supposed to fuse together didn't, which we refer to as a pars interarticularis defect, not much different than cleft lip, cleft palate, or spina bifida. Someone with the pars defect likely has a collagen gene mutation.

In addition to Ehlers-Danlos, Marfan syndrome, Stickler syndrome, OI (osteogenesis imperfecta), pseudoxanthoma elasticum, and many others, dysautonomia is seen frequently. I will describe some differences among the different hypermobility disorders, of which EDS is the Cadillac of the group. With Marfan syndrome, the phenotype is typically the wingspan—it is 1.1 times more than the height. The patient is severely nearsighted, so bad the lens dislocates, known as ectopic lens. He or she gets extreme aortic regurgitation because the valve is too floppy.

A feature of Stickler syndrome, for example, is deafness. That occurs because the ear canal is narrowed, which causes conductive hearing loss, and then the canal fills up with wax, causing more conductive hearing loss. Stickler syndrome gives sensory neuronal hearing loss as well. Osteogenesis imperfecta patients have very high risk of fractures and dozens of fractures at an early age is not uncommon. Those with pseudoxanthoma elasticum have extremely stretchy skin to the point it has been nicknamed chicken skin on one's neck. These patients will not have successful outcomes with plastic surgery.

One may argue the hypermobility spectrum is a normal variant, such a tremendous amount of people have it (most are undiagnosed). My practice has more dysautonomia than any other diagnosis.

But what's more shocking is how difficult it is for patients before they come to me. They've all been to the GP, the emergency room, two orthopedic surgeons, a neurologist, and a neurosurgeon. They've probably been to a psychiatrist. They might have gone to another rheumatologist! I am not reinventing the wheel. This is all in the books! Doctors merely have to read them!

The patients say to me, "Why do you take off my shoes and socks?"

I say, "I have to do a comprehensive exam."

"Well, this is the most comprehensive exam I ever had. Nobody's ever touched my fingers. No one's ever looked at my toes."

I tell them, "A lot of stuff can be learned here." But first you must look. You must know what you are looking at. Many people are told they're crazy. That's probably the number one complaint I get. Even if we pretend they really are crazy, *crazy* is not a diagnosis. They probably have an anxiety disorder or may be bipolar. But they have something treatable. They are not lying; they need the right diagnosis and the right doctor (maybe me).

They're crying. They come in thinking I am another waste of time. I examine them. When I'm with them for an hour and I tell them what they have, they are bawling their eyes out. "You are the first doctor that listened to me. Now you are giving me an answer!" They can't believe it. I guarantee them: 90 percent of my patients are better by 90 percent 100 percent of the time.

## Myositis

Myositis or muscle inflammation causes muscle weakness, not muscle pain. Muscle weakness is very interesting. Eye muscle weakness causes double vision. Esophageal weakness (distal 1/3, striated muscle) may cause trouble swallowing solid foods, but not liquids. As long as the tube is open, the liquids go right down. Shortness of breath happens with intercostal muscle and diaphragm weakness. If those muscles are not working, you can't breathe. The amount of etiologies causing muscle weakness is ubiquitous; however, I will focus on the inflammatory myopathies. I will point out there are common entities that mimic inflammatory myopathies such as hypothyroid or a slow thyroid. My point is one needs a thorough evaluation prior to entertaining anything in the discussion below.

The inflammatory myopathies have a predilection for the proximal muscles, shoulders/deltoid, and hips/quadriceps weakness—the Cadillac of muscle groups, if you will. A more rare myopathy affects elderly men called inclusion body myositis. It causes distal muscle weakness, decreased grip, finger weakness, and atrophy of the forearm. It may be asymmetric, whereas typical inflammatory myopathy are symmetric and proximal. There are several inflammatory myopathies: polymyositis, dermatomyositis, immune-mediated necrotizing myopathy, cancer-related myopathy, juvenile myopa-thy, inclusion body myositis. The list goes on. The typical patient will say they cannot climb stairs anymore or can no longer hold their arms up to wash their hair. I examine them and confirm they're weak. I check blood tests and see their muscle enzyme is elevated. In that case, I may do electro-myography (EMG) and nerve conduction study.

Testing has evolved over the past fifteen years. We now have muscle spe-cific antibodies (MSA). Someone who complains of muscle weakness with a synthetase antibody a JO-1 antibody, EJ, OJ, PL7, PL12, that person has syn-thetase syndrome. Biopsy will reveal inflamed muscle, which we refer to as myopathy related to synthetase syndrome. Such a patient has to be treated very aggressively. The cardinal rule: prevent death from rapidly progressive interstitial lung disease.

Polymyositis and dermatomyositis have similar symmetric proximal muscle weakness with elevated muscle enzyme and an abnormal EMG with classic abnormal muscle biopsy. However, dermatomyositis is asso-ciated with classic rashes—a purple, violaceous rash above the eyes called a heliotrope. Over the neck this is called the shawl sign. Classic skin lesions in dermatomyositis are on the dorsum of joints—crusty, scaly lesions that can mimic psoriasis and are commonly seen on the dorsum of the fingers, the knuckles. (A rash between the knuckles is usually a Lupus rash, whereas a rash on the knuckles is a myositis rash. It can also occur on the elbows and on any dorsal surface. I've seen it on the knee-cap. But you'll typically see it on the knuckles.) It is important to note that a dermatomyositis rash can occur in the absence of muscle weak-ness. This so-called "amyopathic" dermatomyositis. There has been a renaissance in diagnosis and evaluation of dermatomyositis due to the muscle specific antibodies. MI-2 antibody is associated with a straight-forward typically benign phenotype. While MDA-5 is associated with only skin disease no muscle weakness but rapidly progressive interstitial lung disease and poor outcome, often from cancer. NXP-2 is associated with both malignancy and calcium deposit (calcinosis) which is generally untreatable. TIF-1 gamma is highly associated with malignancy in the face of dermatomyositis.

Immune-mediated necrotizing myopathy presents with insidious symmetric proximal muscle weakness with elevated muscle enzymes. However, the muscle biopsy fails to show findings to suggest dermatomyositis or polymyositis, and staining muscle necrosis with minimal inflammatory cells see no immune component. Antibodies SRP and HMG-CoA are of great importance. The SRP-positive patients typically have a worse prognosis and the HMG-CoA reductase antibody patients.

Myositis is a heterogeneous class of diseases causing inflammation of the striated muscle. They can affect anybody of any age and sex. Which muscle is weak and how severe it is will determine the symptom. Those with severe neck muscle weakness will not be able to lift their head off a bed. They can't get up and have no control over it. By and large, people do well when the proper treatment is administered in the appropriate time frame. This doesn't always happen because people don't know to see the right doctor and their regular doctors usually don't know anything. This can cause a long delay in diagnosis which leads to poor outcomes.

The myopathies are interesting because they often overlap with other conditions. By and large, all these autoimmune diseases are more frequent in women than men. Seventy-five percent of my patients are women. Lupus is 10:1 female to male. Rheumatoid arthritis is 4:1 female to male. But I always say, "If you are a man with lupus don't even try to second guess it, because 10:1 is the same as 1,000:10 or 1,000,000:100,000." These are large numbers even though the odds are seemingly small. It's the absolute number that matters. Two of my most ill patients with lupus happen to be elderly men. Always remember: diseases do not read the textbook.

## Scleroderma

There is overlap between myositis and scleroderma. Scleroderma is both inflammatory and fibrotic. This combination makes it unique among the connective tissue diseases. The fibrotic component of disease is responsible for thickening of skin and other organs making soft pliable materials virtually turn to cardboard. Patients with an increase in dermal collagen will end up having hidebound skin, like leather. That's what people think of with scleroderma. However, all organs may be involved, the most ominous being the lungs. The whole body gets that way—blood vessels, lungs, thyroid.

If lungs become leatherlike, it doesn't matter if they're inflamed. They were not functioning properly. Restrictive lung disease will occur and is often progressive. The bowels are often involved. Lack of motion in the small bowel can lead to bacterial overgrowth which causes refractory diarrhea, while lack of motion in the large intestine or colon leads to constipation that is hard to treat. Itching is a common feature of scleroderma, possibly because of calcium deposition. This is very difficult to treat. Patients with scleroderma frequently have a slow thyroid and often testicular dysfunction in men.

There are many types of scleroderma: systemic scleroderma, limited scleroderma (formally called CREST), localized, linear (calcinosis, Raynaud, esophageal dysmotility, sclerodactyly, and telangiectasia).

CREST is associated with the anticentromere antibody, while the systemic sclerosis is associated with the antitopoisomerase antibody, or scl-70 antibody. These associations are not set in stone and either disease can have either antibody. The importance of the antibodies is the association of pulmonary hypertension or the associated interstitial lung disease.

The important thing is to save lives and improve quality of life. Decades ago, death in scleroderma was caused by hypertensive renal crisis, extremely high blood pressure, and concurrent kidney failure. With the advent of angiotensin convertase inhibitors (ace), there is no more death. Problem eliminated.

Captopril, the first ace inhibitor, is FDA approved for high blood pressure at 50 milligrams and heart failure at 100 milligrams. In scleroderma it is used as high as 800 milligrams/day, and it works well. No one should die from scleroderma renal crisis anymore.

In the next leading cause of death associated with scleroderma, lung disease, anticentromere antibodies are associated with pulmonary hypertension while anti-SCL 70 antibody is associated with interstitial lung disease. Be mindful: myositis can overlap with scleroderma not uncommonly with or without antibodies. These patients are at more risk of progressive interstitial lung disease. Currently interstitial lung disease is not adequately treatable and without heart lung transplant will lead to death. Several medications have indications for interstitial lung disease in the setting of scleroderma; however, in reality the outcomes are not good. Conversely, pulmonary artery hypertension has become quite manageable.

I am appalled insurance companies will not approve proper medication unless excessive heart testing, namely a right heart catheterization is performed. This is not a walk in the park and it is very expensive, however the cost analysis favors the drug company hoping the numbers will fall below their threshold to pay for the medication.

Let us discuss the medications. There are three classes of the phosphodiesterase inhibitor sildenafil—the same product as Viagra. The dosing is different, the names are different but it is the same product. The exact mechanism of action is not known; however, it tends to open the blood vessels and allow more blood through to the lungs. Endothelial cell antagonist, the lining of the blood vessels, or endothelial cells, is comprised by smooth muscle, which is aided by this class of medication. And finally, the prostacyclin switch: here, a very potent vasodilator is added to the first two medications. It's a game changer and patients are living much longer.

Another interesting complication in the scleroderma population is the deposition of hydroxyapatite. This is essentially bone which deposits under the skin and other places. It can be very painful and not treatable.

In one patient the hydroxyapatite was so excessive, pieces the size of toothpicks were falling through the skin like shampoo running out of the jar. Sadly that was the one day I did not have a camera handy.

## Raynaud Syndrome

Raynaud syndrome is a disease to itself with manifestations that are limited to lack of blood to the affected extremity. While Raynaud's phenomena may be associated with scleroderma or any other connective tissue disease, an acceptable definition for Raynaud's is a reversible spasm of the arteries going into the digits or the hands or the nose, and lasting five to sixty minutes. It is frequently seen with a triple phase color response: white-blue-red. Blood stops entering the finger, and it immediately turns white. After sitting around losing oxygen from that blood the color becomes bluish purple, when the closed artery opens fresh oxygenated blood rushes in and causes a red flush. This phenomenon can occur virtually anywhere, but it typically happens in cold weather or from emotional stress and affects the fingers, toes, ears, and nose. Untreated this can be dangerous as distal ischemia may lead to death of bone, loss of bone, loss of soft tissue, and deep infections. Many treatments exist that are partially useful. The best treatment is likely a PDE 5 inhibitor such as sildenafil; however it is not FDA approved for this treatment.

Scleroderma and myositis are frequently seen together. I met a woman in the hospital a while back whose antinuclear antibodies (ANA) test was positive, very high. Her pericardium was filled with fluid. I looked at her hands and said, "Gosh, you know, you look like you have scleroderma or myositis." She had Gottron lesions, her CPK was 2,000, whereas normal is up to 150. I said, "You have dermatomyositis." She ended up getting an MRI of her low back or buttocks because of an X-ray showing something irregular. It turned out that she had muscle edema all throughout the butt. She got a muscle biopsy to confirm her diagnosis. The patient became depressed, refused treatment, left the hospital and attempted suicide by jumping off the Ben Franklin Bridge. The patient was then brought to a hospital again. By this time she was doing worse and the physicians in Philadelphia called to tell me the skin biopsy was done and it showed she had scleroderma in addition to dermatomyositis.

Now, did she have scleroderma with myositis or myositis with scleroderma? It is pretty irrelevant. The patient had lost two fingers before I was even called. When I met her, there was necrosis. Prior to rheumatology being involved in this case the other physicians wanted to amputate all of her fingers. They did not recognize digital ischemia that was associated with her underlying disease, while they speculated there were infections there was no proof of such.

There is no treatment for skin tightening. Fortunately people don't often die of skin tightness. However, the worse the skin is, the more likely the patient is to have internal organ disease.

The best test, above and beyond examination of the patients and of antibodies, is called nailfold capillaroscopy. I put mineral oil right at the cuticle and, using an ophthalmoscope or a nailfold capillaroscopy scope, I can actually see the capillaries. If they look normal, the patient may not have anything. If they are abnormal, dilated, bushy, or contain dropout of capillary loops, the person likely has scleroderma or myositis, although abnormal findings are seen in lupus and other connective-tissue diseases. If they're abnormal, you have a serious problem, and it needs further evaluation immediately.

Most people actually do well, just like my lupus patients. The published data shows all lupus patients dying. I've got dozens of lupus patients with terrible kidney disease. If they follow my directions and I am allowed to administer proper drugs, they're not dying and they're not on dialysis. They're having babies. But they need to see a doctor who knows what he or she is doing.

## Polymyalgia Rheumatica

Polymyalgia rheumatica (PMR) is common, more so in elderly white people. It does not occur under the age of about fifty. But anybody over fifty with pain and morning stiffness in the neck, shoulders, hip, and buttocks/ proximal girdle pain, probably has that condition. Occasionally it is confused with rheumatoid arthritis due to small joint involvement of the hands and feet. However, in polymyalgia rheumatica, the rheumatoid factor is negative.

The typical picture is a seventy-year-old who reports, "For the last year, I'm stuck in bed; I can't get out. It takes me two hours to get moving."

I say, "Okay, I know what you have."

He says, "What are you talking about? I haven't been here thirty seconds."

I say, "Look, I know what you have." They look at me like I'm crazy. I ask Denise, "Would you tell him what he has?"

She says, "You have Polymyalgia rheumatica."

"Well, how do you know?"

I know because I diagnose it once a week. It's easily treatable, and very gratifying for me as the physician to see such improvement in such a short amount of time. The problem with this condition, if left untreated or if treated without follow-up, is that it can relapse in the form of giant cell arteritis, or temporal arteritis. That is vasculitis of the large vessels, historically the temporal arteries, which can lead to blindness, stroke, or death. Death can be prevented by diagnosing giant cell arteritis and by giving high-dose IV steroids immediately.

Inflammation is defined by redness, heat, swelling, and warmth. But inflammation could be from an infection or cancer. It's for me to sort out that a patient doesn't have cancer or infections.

That comes from the history, from talking to patients. You can get so much by talking to patients. But you have to interrogate them. I am really an interrogator. A lot of my patients say I'm cutting them off. But I say, "No, I'm asking what I need to know." I find that when I'm having extended conversations with patients, every now and again they'll say something like, "Well, does it matter that when I was younger, I used to get mouth sores every third Tuesday of every July?"

"Oh, my God, yes, that's huge!" I'll say. "That's very important." And it is. The crucial thing is to know how to put the clues together and to know what to ask. Nobody thinks to call a rheumatologist. I diagnosed a lady while I was in the gym once. She had been in the hospital for ten days and her treating physicians called everybody except rheumatology. I was able to diagnose her in the gym because I knew what questions to ask, and I knew what her answers meant.

I have now diagnosed about 1,500 people with polymyalgia rheumatica, but I've been burned about fifteen times. Out of the fifteen, one had cancer, one had an infection, and thirteen had psoriatic arthritis. My contention, which I am writing a paper on, is that, based on my findings, if you see a patient with polymyalgia rheumatica who doesn't follow a classic course right away, you need to suspect psoriatic arthritis.

## An Update on Gout

Krystexxa is a uricase inhibitor which converts uric acid to allantoin. Some people do not have a uricase gene, thus they are unable to break down uric acid. This medication works for 70 percent of patients; it lowers uric acid to 0. However, due to tolerance or immunogenicity, it is rendered disabled in about a third of patients. And if you use certain antibody-blocking drugs, usually methotrexate, it can work 85 percent of the time. The drug is extremely useful; however it is often not necessary due to existing conventional treatments.

Even though I've tried the drug, I believe that if you treat gout properly, you don't need it. If you kill everybody with a gun, you don't need a nuclear bomb.

Now, due to insurance-company greed, I've been forced to fight for people who need Krystexxa—which costs more than $30,000 per treatment—in spite of the failure of the highest dose of allopurinol or patients who could not use it safely. There is no data to support combining allopurinol with uloric except in my recent article. Well, I combined it, and I was able to get people's uric acid down to 3.0. At 3.0, they can eat and drink, with no exception, all day long and still improve.

But no data mentions it. I am writing up the three cases showing that it's safe and it worked. In the United States, gout is treated terribly. Most people don't realize that to control most gout patients allopurinol in a dose of 400 mg up to 800 mg may be necessary and most doctors are not comfortable prescribing anything other than 100 mg or 300 mg. Please do not ask me to explain why this is. I have no idea. Gout patients are clearly underdosed, and undertreated. Sadly they do not do well with one of the most treatable diseases.

Patients on allopurinol say, "Oh, I'm on gout medicine; it sucks. Look, my blood is normal." I look at their blood. The normal uric acid level is from 3.0 to 8.0. But for a severe gout patient, anything over 5.0 is too high. If someone's level is 6.6, the lab says the person is normal, but that person is actually doing terrible.

Somebody like myself recognizes that everybody on 300 milligrams of allopurinol has uric acid between 7.0 and 8.0, which, sure, is better than 15.0. But it still sucks, and the people are getting worse. You have to add uloric because they can't tolerate Krystexxa. When you add uloric, the uric acid drops significantly. I don't see the rocket science here. But since nobody thought of it, it's on me.

No insurance will cover the combination. The company will say it's not indicated. When I write the paper and the company inevitably denies the treatment, I'm going to say, "Here is the article. And by the way, I wrote it."

That's the only reason I'm now interested in writing for publication. When I fight on the phone, being published gives me much more ammunition. The academicians have five hundred papers; I have twenty. But the academicians don't fight anybody because they don't see patients.

## The Patient Walk-Through

Say someone who comes in to see me reports pain. First, I ask myself, *Is it arthritic or is it unrelated?* Once I have classified it as arthritis, I look at the arthritis by the pattern of joints—small and large.

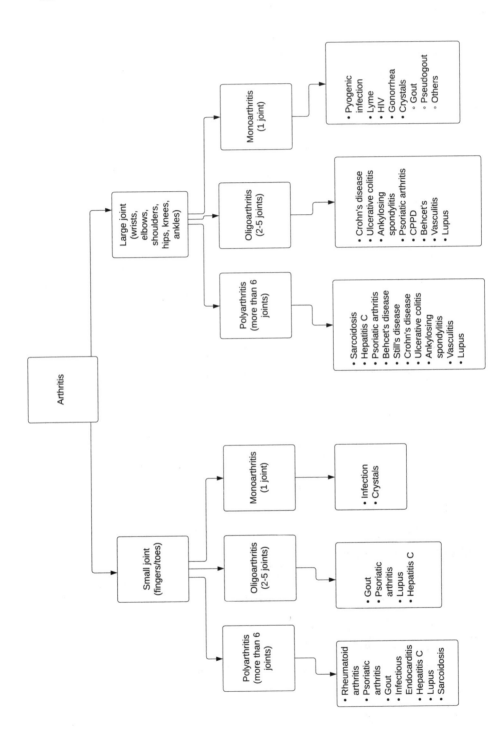

On the left are the small joints: fingers and toes. And on the right are the large joints: wrists, elbows, shoulders, hips, knees, ankles. These are further classified into polyarthritis (meaning more than six joints), oligoarthritis (2–5 joints), and monoarthritis (1 joint).

We look at arthritis as inflammatory or noninflammatory.

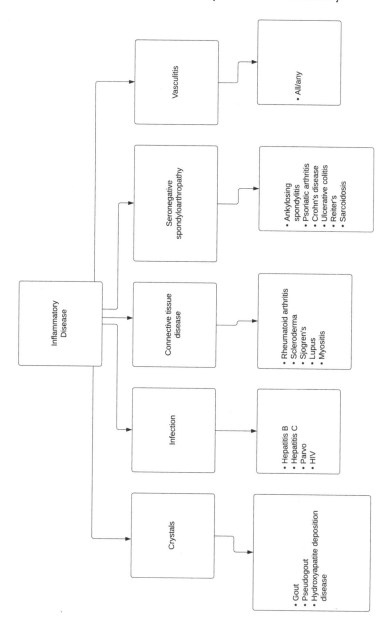

Under inflammatory are five categories:

- Crystals: gout, pseudogout, hydroxyapatite deposition disease.
- Infection: hepatitis B, C, HIV, parvo, infectious endocarditis.
- Connective tissue diseases: rheumatoid arthritis, lupus, Sjogren syndrome, scleroderma, myositis.
- Seronegative spondyloarthropathy (SPA) ankylosing spondylitis, psoriatic arthritis, inflammatory bowel disease (IBD), Crohn disease, and ulcerative colitis. Under that is Reiter syndrome, also known as reactive arthritis. And then under that is sarcoidosis. And rarely Whipple's or Behcet's, too.
- Vasculitis

Many of these diseases overlap.

The following example depicts the overlap of three diseases. In this modified Venn diagram, the top left is rheumatoid arthritis, the top right is lupus, and the bottom is Sjogren syndrome.

Rheumatoid arthritis involves joints; Raynaud syndrome; sicca symptoms, which really mean dry eyes and dry mouth; pulmonary or lung manifestations; increased rheumatoid factor (ANA) positive and 25 percent; and DS DNA negative. Lupus involves joints, rash, sicca symptoms, ANA elevation, DNA positive, rheumatoid factor positive and about 25 percent, cyclic citrullinated peptide (CCP) negative, Raynaud syndrome, pulmonary manifestation, and cytopenia. Sjogren syndrome involves positive ANA, rheumatoid factor, Sjogren syndrome A (SSA), Sjogren syndrome B (SSB), negative CCP, negative DNA, Raynaud's phenomena/disease, pulmonary manifestation, cytopenia, joints, and sicca symptoms (dry eyes and dry mouth).

The UCTD listed at the bottom stands for unspecified connective-tissue disease. If someone doesn't fulfill the criteria for any one disease but definitely has something related to connective tissue, it's merely an unspecified connective-tissue disease.

This is by no means encyclopedic, though I use this outline when patients tell me they have lupus. I usually want to explain to them that they have arthritis and have ANA, but they can have any one of these three afflictions, or ten others.

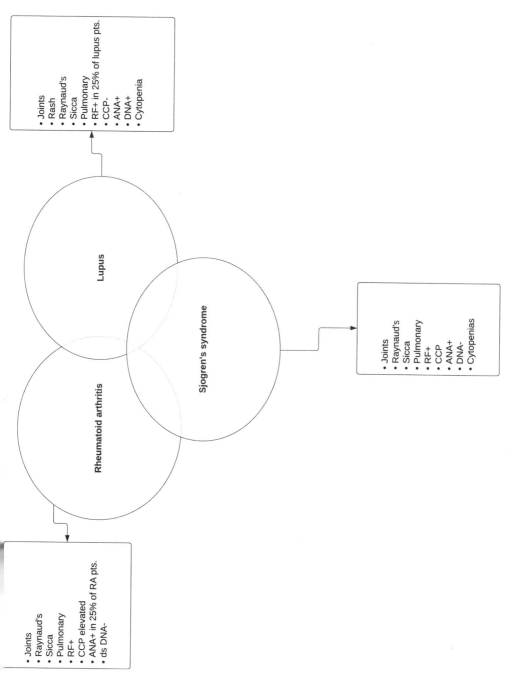

Lupus
- Joints
- Rash
- Raynaud's
- Sicca
- Pulmonary
- RF+ in 25% of lupus pts.
- CCP-
- ANA+
- DNA+
- Cytopenia

Sjogren's syndrome
- Joints
- Raynaud's
- Sicca
- Pulmonary
- RF+
- CCP
- ANA+
- DNA-
- Cytopenias

Rheumatoid arthritis
- Joints
- Raynaud's
- Sicca
- Pulmonary
- RF+
- CCP elevated
- ANA+ in 25% of RA pts.
- ds DNA-

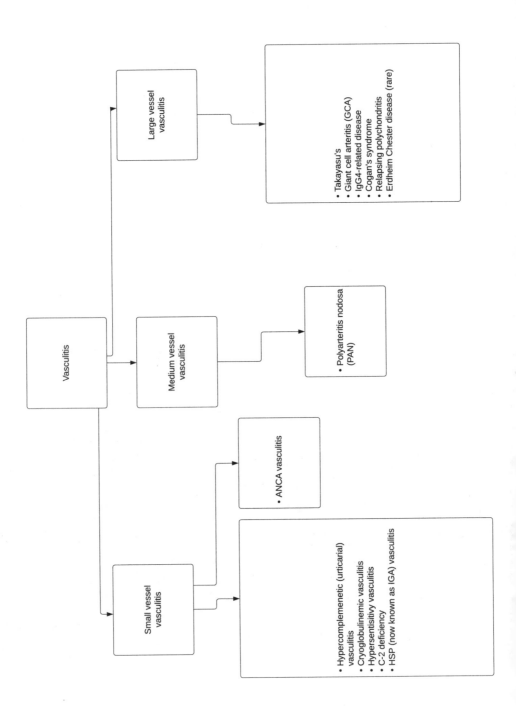

We classify vasculitis as small-vessel vasculitis (SVV), medium-vessel vasculitis (MVV), and large-vessel vasculitis (LVV). The three are very distinct from each other.

Under small-vessel vasculitis are hypocomplementemic urticarial vasculitis, cryoglobulinemic vasculitis, hypersensitivity vasculitis, C-2 deficiency, and Henoch-Scönlein purpura (HSP), now known as Immunoglobulin A (IgA) vasculitis. Also, the abbreviation ANCA is Anti-Neutrophilic Cytoplasmic Autoantibody vasculitis, which usually presents as a small-vessel vasculitis.

Refer to the beautiful chart of vasculitis on the previous page.

ANCA vasculitis has its own identity. If a patient is ANCA-positive, you then need to get ELISA testing for the specific antibody MPO, or myeloperoxidase, or PR-3, proteinase-3. PR-3 positivity in the right clinical scenario used to be called Wegener disease but is now called granulomatosis polyangiitis. MPO is associated most commonly with microscopic polyangiitis, renal limited vasculitis, and eosinophilic granulomatous polyangiitis. PR-3 is most commonly associated with what was formally called Wegener's granulomatosis. These definitions are not set in stone. Many individuals will have both antibodies positive and a protean manifestation, PIP.

If you get a patient with hemorrhage from the lungs and kidneys at the same time, that's pulmonary renal syndrome. You have to recognize it right away and treat it quickly. I added that on the P-ANCA. In addition to inflammatory bowel disease, lupus, and sarcoidosis, cocaine is a culprit. Cocaine-induced vasculitis is actually quite common.

On the other side of the small-vessel vasculitis spectrum, I have systemic lupus erythematosus (SLE), or lupus; rheumatoid arthritis; cancer; and lymphoma. Why? Connective-tissue diseases can cause vasculitis. Malignancies can give vasculitis. So lupus, rheumatoid arthritis, and all the other diseases listed can have vasculitis.

You are getting the picture that vasculitis is a very large category! It's far more common than the other categories. Each category of disease has the most-common and the worst-case type. The most common in this category

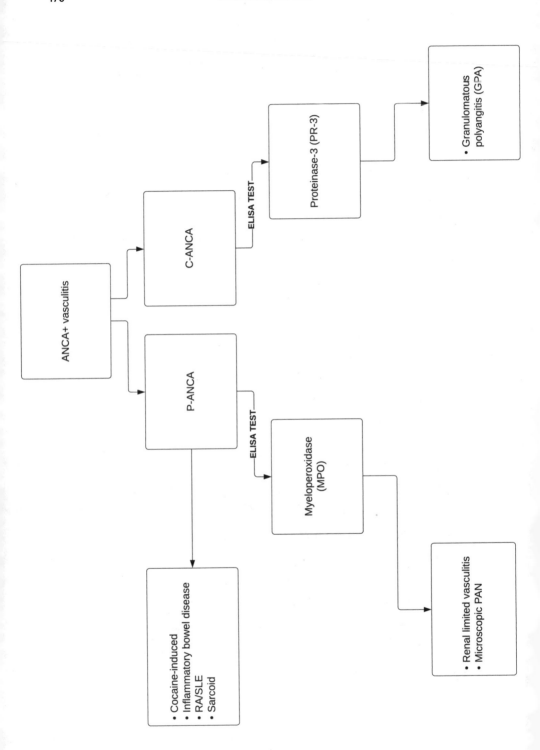

is hypersensitivity vasculitis, which is often caused by an allergy to a drug of some sort. It usually goes away. More ominous would be if somebody has a cancer that happens to show up as a vasculitis. That person's not going to do well.

The Cadillac of medium-vessel vasculitis is polyarteritis nodosa, or PAN. The medium vessels include the arteries to the kidneys, stomach, and bowels. They're referred to as the celiac arteries, superior mesenteric arteries, and renal arteries, which create infarction in the kidneys, gut, and bowel. If somebody has small-vessel vasculitis of the gut, bowel wall edema and pain will be present. If somebody gets medium-vessel vasculitis of the gut, that person will actually create infarction in the bowel and need resection and surgery. This condition spares the lungs and must be differentiated on occasion from fibromuscular dysplasia which has a rather benign course.

Large-vessel vasculitis, as stated, involves the largest of the blood vessels and any malfunction of the largest blood vessels. Dissection, aneurysm, and inflammation can all lead to hemorrhage and rapid death.

The primary large-vessel vasculitic diseases are Takayasu arteritis, which affects young women, and GCA, or giant cell arteritis, which is usually in older white men. Giant cell arteritis normally affects the temporal arteries in the scalp. One can have extracranial disease, which involves any branch of the aorta.

The following conditions can all manifest as large vessel vasculitis. While they are all unique, they should never be forgotten. They include IgG4-related disease, Behcet's, Cogan's, Erdheim-Chester, relapsing polychondritis, and retroperitoneal fibrosis. People with IgG4-related disease get what is referred to as the *sausage pancreas*, where the pancreas shrinks up. There may be inflammatory changes of the gallbladder, swollen glands in and around the face, the parotid gland, the thyroid gland. Cases of cranial nerve involvement, the orbits, and more have been described. This condition would be diagnosed by biopsy. Cogan syndrome occurs in the setting of sensorineural hearing loss and visual disturbance. Relapsing polychondritis involves inflammation of cartilage, such as at the top of the ear or the top of the nose. Cardiac pulmonary and ocular involvement are common. Behcet's disease is commonly manifested by the involvement of mouth and genital ulcers, pulmonary artery aneurysms, and several skin lesions, erythema nodosa the most common. Finally, the rarity Erdheim-Chester disease is characterized by histiocytic infiltrates in addition to large vessel vasculitis. Long bones are affected causing pain near the wrists and ankles.

You might think, *The category is vasculitis*. A lot of these diseases present in different fashions. If I see somebody with inflammatory arthritis, there is an applicable category called fibrocartilaginous diseases. Under that is IgG4. In fact, I think it's the only disease in that category. As discussed, it can also present as a large-vessel vasculitis. When I say one disease "presents" as another disease, it means the same disease can mimic another disease.

Here is an example. A patient could be stuck in the hospital for a month with fevers and nobody knows what's wrong. The person is not complaining of arthritis or arthritic symptoms; the patient just feels lousy. When a doctor orders testing and finds out that the aorta is inflamed or enlarged, all of a sudden IgG4 would go on the large vessel vasculitis possibilities or differential diagnosis. The best way to diagnose this is by fluorodeoxyglucose positron emission tomography (FDG-PET) scan. However, note that the insurance companies often deny the test even though it is the standard of care!

Most of these diseases are heterogeneous meaning they look different all the time. A simple example is lupus. The disease can be severe lupus, which people want to classify as kidney lupus, and non-life-threatening lupus, which involves skin or joints. Some experts want to subcategorize instead of just lupus.

The inflammatory myopathy chart is the nomenclature for the inflammatory muscle diseases: dermatomyositis, immune mediated necrotizing myopathy, and synthetase syndrome. The one I don't have listed here is inclusion body myositis, or ICBM. (ICBM is dangerous but rare—I've seen perhaps two cases in my life. It is easily recognizable.)

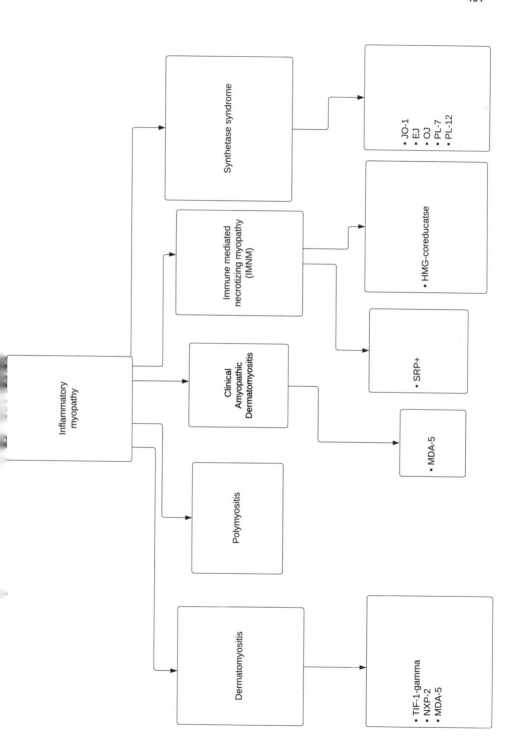

As I said, the new thing that's gone on in myositis diagnosis and treatment is the discovery of all these antibodies. But the commonality among inflammatory myopathy patients is weakness. By and large, they have proximal muscle weakness: shoulders and neck and hips (as opposed to inclusion body myositis, which manifests forearm and calf weakness). Proximal muscle weakness is symmetric, whereas inclusion-body weakness is asymmetric. The differentiation of these is important because, generally, dermatomyositis is easily treatable, and it's monocyclic—it goes away after proper treatment.

Myositis-specific antibodies associated with dermatomyositis are listed: TIF-1-gamma, highly associated with malignancy, NXP-2, highly associated with malignancy or refractory calcinosis, and MDA-5 associated with clinical amyopathic dermatomyositis, rapidly progressive interstitial lung disease, and malignancy.

The immune mediated necrotizing myopathy group is differentiated into two categories: SRP-positive and HMG-CoA reductase. The SRP-positive people do poorly, and they require very aggressive therapy. The HMG-CoA reductase people do relatively well, and they indeed require aggressive therapy as well. Another group of IMNM patients are unspecified, and we don't know what they represent.

Synthetase syndrome is unique because it is, for lack of a better definition, an inflammatory myopathy on biopsy with interstitial lung disease in conjunction with the synthetase antibodies, JO-1, which makes up a third of the cases; PL-7; EJ; OJ; and PL-12.

If a patient has muscle weakness, two things need to occur: get a muscle biopsy to confirm what's going on. At the same time, you have to order the panel of antibody tests.

*Phenotype* is what the doctor sees. *Genotype* is the genetic constitution. I have a patient who is weak. The only phenotype that suggests the patient has dermatomyositis is the classic rash. Otherwise, the biopsy may confirm a diagnosis. Often, the treatment is empiric. The results of testing may not come back for several days or weeks.

What causes these diseases is unknown. People often have a genetic predisposition as many diseases tend to have genetic tendencies.

What I tell people—which is the real answer—is that you inherit a genetic barcode. You get a billion pieces from mom and a billion pieces from dad. If you are inheriting the same barcode, you have the same genetic predisposition as your parents have. Whether you come in contact with the unknown environmental stimulus, viral or otherwise, will determine whether yours is going to turn on, so to speak. We just don't know how this works. It is one of the most fascinating things about these diseases, but it's also one of the worst because the people that are *not* in this field are feckless and forget rheumatology exists. We may not fully understand these diseases, but we partially understand a small piece!

## The Mind of a Rheumatologist

All of the foregoing shows how I work through a person in pain. Is the pain arthritic? If so, is the arthritis inflamed? Is it just wear and tear? If it's inflammatory, is the arthritis small, medium, or large? Does it occur in one, several, or many joints? If it is noninflammatory, that's osteoarthritis, OA. Under the OA classification, is primary or secondary. Primary means wear and tear, whereas secondary involves something such as hemochromatosis. A condition, calcium pyrophosphate arthropathy, is under both subcategories of inflammatory and noninflammatory and causes cartilage damage, as opposed to wear and tear, which is secondary osteoarthritis.

This is how the mind of a rheumatologist works: All of these diseases have commonalities—joint disease, pain, swelling, arthritis, and the like. If a patient come to a doctor's office with a swollen joint, the person's affliction is bound to be in one of those six categories. That is why rheumatology is the field of orthopedics *without* surgery. But orthopedic doctors have never heard of any of them. They're not trained to understand and diagnose the problems, just like I'm not trained in how to put on casts and how to operate on a bad joint to replace it. They're just trained on how to cut out the bad stuff and replace it with better material. Orthopedics is surgery of the bones, plain and simple. A rheumatologist is the doctor who, based on history, physical exam, and analysis of joint fluid, will come up with a diagnosis and treatment plan that does not require surgery.

Do not be misled by the term *bone-on-bone*. If you hear this term, someone is trying to coerce you into surgery. A proper injection may buy you six months or more of pain-free living. And it can be repeated if necessary. Not all patients are surgical candidates; they should not be forgotten.

## What's new in Rheumatoid Arthritis?

Rheumatoid arthritis is a systemic inflammatory condition with a predilection for the small joints. While it commonly presents as polyarthritis, it may present as oligoarticular, monoarthritis, and occasionally palindromic and lead into rheumatoid arthritis. Small joints in a symmetric pattern are the norm, however large joints are involved with regularity. Extra-articular manifestations include rheumatoid nodules and rheumatoid lung disease. The most common is pleurisy. The worst case scenario is interstitial lung disease or lung cancer, rarely seen rheumatoid vasculitis. Rheumatoid arthritis can often be misdiagnosed as gout or psoriatic arthritis.

To make a definite diagnosis of rheumatoid arthritis, I would not rely on research criteria because that is not meant for diagnosis. The criteria are meant for homogenizing groups of people for clinical trials.

If a person has a positive rheumatoid factor and a positive CCP antibody with everything else negative or normal and small joint symmetric arthritis with or without nodules, that person probably would have rheumatoid arthritis. Until you exclude hepatitis C, cryoglobulins, and monoclonal immunoglobulin deposition diseases, I suggest those assessments are done prior to giving the official diagnosis of rheumatoid arthritis. I recommend, if the rheumatoid factor and CCP are both negative, checking the 14-3-3 eta protein. This is more specific than the other two markers. If those three studies are positive with a symmetric small joint arthritis, the sensitivity and specificity is likely 95 percent.

What other organs are involved in rheumatoid arthritis? Most common would be subcutaneous nodules; however, the biopsy showing palisading layers of neutrophils can be seen in other benign nodules in other conditions, such as juvenile arthritis. The finding of nodules portends a worse prognosis, and, interestingly, it likely has a different pathogenic mechanism, as methotrexate, the gold standard for treatment, makes the nodules worse. Plaquenil can shrink the nodules, and biologic therapy has not been shown to improve nodules. Thus, akin to psoriatic arthritis versus psoriasis skin disease, there may be a difference in pathophysiology.

Although the cause of rheumatoid arthritis is not known, genetic HLA-DR4 and hormonal factors are in play. Clearly, rheumatoid arthritis affects women more than men and 50 percent of pregnant women go into remission during pregnancy. Some are actually cured and never have a disease recurrence. Unlike lupus, rheumatoid arthritis is typically not affected by the sun. Psoriatic arthritis and psoriasis are typically improved by the sun.

Rheumatoid lung involvement is quite common. Interstitial lung disease, rheumatoid nodules, and pleurisy may all antedate the onset of joint disease, and having a positive rheumatoid factor with any of those lung issues is not a guarantee of RA, as lupus and others can do the same. Pleuritic disease may antedate the actual arthritis. If the rheumatoid factor is very high, it makes the rheumatoid diagnosis a bit more likely, and the rheumatoid factor can be followed for changes in disease activity, unlike the ANA in lupus and unlike the DNA in lupus that is not involving a proliferative renal lesion.

Over the past twenty-five years, many novel therapies have come along to treat rheumatoid arthritis. The gold standard over the past fifty years has remained methotrexate.

Prior to biologic therapy, the gold standard treatment would include a combination of Plaquenil, sulfasalazine, methotrexate, or a combination of methotrexate and gold, oral or intramuscular, oil-based or water-based. The only drugs previously shown to have good effect clinically were methotrexate gold and Penicillamine. The latter had too many side effects and was never a mainstay in treatment.

Current treatments including TNF inhibitors, IL-1, IL-6, IL-17, and JAK inhibitors (the three currently approved by the FDA), along with low-dose steroids and continuous ongoing methotrexate have changed the playing field from one-third of people crippled to virtually no one. The true nonresponders, in my estimation, would indicate that the diagnosis is incorrect rather than that the drugs don't work. I think spending more money at that point by prescribing any other treatments or me-too drugs is frivolous, as we already have eliminated NSAIDs for the treatment of rheumatoid arthritis, along with most of the associated GI bleeds.

Rheumatoid arthritis is a vastly complex multisystem disease with a predilection for symmetric small-joint synovitis, able to affect virtually any part of the body with various genetic predispositions and toxic environmental triggers. We now find ourselves with near perfection in remission in a large majority of these patients.

It is extremely important to make the correct diagnosis so the correct treatment can be achieved. This is done through careful history and physical examination, proper assessment of differential diagnosis, evaluation of lab data, X-rays, other imaging modalities, and reconciliation of a plan tailored for the patient. Examples of such a plan include the use of B cell blockade in rheumatoid arthritis with concurrent cryoglobulinemia and abatacept, which happens to be T-cell costimulator Orencia, in a patient with rheumatoid arthritis who may have autoantibodies to lupus.

In summary, don't miss the diagnosis. Try to tailor the treatment to the patient.

You should not forget rheumatoid vasculitis. If a chronic untreated rheumatoid patient shows up with ulcers on hands and feet with infarctions, that could signify Raynaud syndrome and overlap syndrome, but don't forget that with a high rheumatoid factor that could be rheumatoid arthritis with vasculitis, treated as vasculitis with cyclophosphamide.

Rheumatoid arthritis, when viewed as a small-joint symmetric polyarthritis, can be confused with viruses, including zika, chikungunya, acute

Lyme disease, HIV, hepatitis B, and hepatitis C, to name a few. Rheumatoid mimics can be seen in arthritis from COVID-19 as well. Other mimics include spondyloarthropathies, not limited to but including ankylosing spondylitis, psoriatic arthritis, Crohn colitis, ulcerative colitis, reactive arthritis or Reiter syndrome, sarcoidosis, Behcet's disease, celiac disease, and Whipple disease. They may all give an arthritis that mimics rheumatoid arthritis.

Cardiac involvement may be present as well. One can have rheumatoid nodules in the conduction system or the valves; or pericardial disease, hoarseness, dysarthria, and swallowing and breathing dysfunction could occur due to cricoid arthritis or rheumatoid nodules in the upper respiratory system. Rheumatoid arthritis typically does not give a primary glomerulonephritis or interstitial cystitis; however, the overlap between rheumatoid arthritis and Sjogren syndrome can give a picture of renal tubular acidosis and interstitial cystitis—rarely glomerular disease—and the overlap of rheumatoid arthritis and lupus can give membranous nephropathy or glomerular nephritis. Chronic rheumatoid arthritis in the pure state can lead to amyloidosis rarely seen in this era, though it should be recognized.

What about what one would call true rheumatoid-factor-negative rheumatoid arthritis, including CCP and 14-3-3 eta? Some of the patients in this group may have polymyalgia rheumatica, and younger patients may actually have vasculitic diseases, perhaps Kawasaki disease. Lymphomas and leukemias are seen frequently as symmetric arthritis and may create problems in the differential diagnoses seen for multiple myeloma and other monoclonal immune globulin deposition diseases.

Regarding treatments, some rheumatologists believe in using steroids, while others don't. Some believe in starting with high steroid doses and weaning off. However, the end result is typically a combination of methotrexate and TNF inhibitor. All TNF inhibitors work better with combination methotrexate.

Methotrexate blocks antibodies that may cause lupus-like reactions or autoantibodies. The combination is indisputably better than giving either drug alone. JAK inhibitors, which are small molecules, and the JAK stat pathway incudes JAK 1, JAK 2, JAK 3, and TYK. These small molecules block intracellular proinflammatory cytokines in large amounts, while tocilizumab works on or binds only interleukin-6. Belimumab (blyss inhibitor), adalimumab (anti-TNF), infliximab (anti-TNF), and abatacept (CTLA4/tcell co-stimulation inhibitor) block T-cells. Saphnelo blocks interferon (INF). The small molecules tend to block combinations of various interleukins and INF. Although this may be practically good in terms of reducing inflammation, it has created black-box warnings for heart attacks and thrombosis. I am leery of the class, although the drugs have shown promise, albeit not of first-line quality.

Abatacept CTLA-4 inhibitor, tocilizumab, interleukin-6 inhibitor, rituximab A, and B-cell depletor are all great drugs in rheumatoid arthritis, but the current standard would be TNF inhibitor with methotrexate. In case of failure, one can determine on a case-by-case basis what is the smartest option. An example would be a rheumatoid patient with cryoglobulins who should go on rituximab due to the blocking of the B cells. The same goes for a rheumatoid-Sjogren overlap. We need to look out for tocilizumab-inducted hyperlipemia or colon perforation and be mindful of patients with diverticular disease prior to starting treatment. We should also be mindful of those with lupus overlap and try to favor B-cell depletion or CTLA-4 inhibition rather than TNF inhibitor.

# CHAPTER 11
# ORTHOPEDICS FOR DUMMIES

Every item in the following list should be treated by a rheumatologist before anyone else. (However, there are exceptional orthopedic surgeons and terrible rheumatologists, so never say *never*, and never say *always*.) Here are the symptoms:

- Hand and wrist pain
- Foot and ankle pain
- Elbow and shoulder pain
- Hip and knee pain
- Neck and low-back pain
- Arthritis
- Tendonitis
- Bursitis
- Spinal stenosis
- Carpal tunnel
- Trigger fingers
- Fasciitis

Everything I wrote in this book pertains to what I see and treat daily. I estimate that "orthopedic" issues make up fifty to sixty percent of what I do.

By and large, family doctors, ER docs, and urgent-care places are programmed to send the work to orthopedics. But *all patients with joint pain should go to a rheumatologist.* You could argue that there are not enough capable rheumatologists, and you would be correct. Orthopedic surgeons outnumber rheumatologists significantly.

About 6,500 rheumatologists are in the United States, only 5,000 of which are in clinical practice. At the same time, orthopedic surgeons number about 25,000. In my county, for example, are two full-time rheumatologists, whereas the orthopedic practice down the street has sixteen orthopedic surgeons. All the work incorrectly goes to orthopedic surgeons.

A swollen knee almost never needs surgery. The fluid needs to be removed and analyzed by a rheumatologist looking for crystals (for gout, pseudogout, oxalosis, and more). Lipid (or fat) in synovial fluid may diagnose a fracture before the surgeon can find it, or pancreatic disease. Finding blood in the joint (hemarthrosis) can represent not only a football injury but gout, cancer, and more! Blood is phlogistic—it incites inflammation.) If the knee does need surgery, you can treat it conservatively first. Conservative treatment would be better done by a nonsurgeon trained in the nonsurgical management of the swollen knee—or the painful shoulder, back pain, heel pain, Achilles pain, carpal tunnel symptoms, or locking finger, a.k.a. trigger finger. That would be a rheumatologist, *not* an orthopedic.

What will happen to the patients not sent to a rheumatologist (which is most patients)? One of three things will occur: They will be sent to the physical-therapy location in the orthopedic surgeon's own office, which will make the problem worse. Perhaps orthopedists will drain the knee or inject steroids. Regardless, the orthopedist will either knowingly perform the wrong procedure or is incompetent. It sadly doesn't work too often, and the patient's surgery is unnecessary. They are told nothing else worked and they have to have surgery. Or, option three, orthopedic surgeons inappropriately resort to arthroscopy. If that doesn't work, they can say, "Oh, well, you need the knee replaced."

On the other hand, if a patient comes to me with a swollen knee, I drain it. I take the synovial fluid to the polarizing microscope and diagnose the knee based on what I see, gout, pseudogout, inflammation. The presence of lipid droplets or fat in the synovial fluid may be indicative of a fracture or pancreatic process.

There is a higher risk of getting unnecessary surgery if patients don't go through a very well-trained rheumatologist. We treat joints better—but perhaps I'm the exception. Many people who have trained in the last five to ten years are not well-trained at joint aspiration or injection, I do not know why. It's sad to see. Rheumatologists are supposed to drain and look at synovial fluid, and they do not know how. They don't know what they're looking for. Like so many aspects of medicine, the paradigm has turned upside down in the last fifteen years. Any newly swollen knee or other joint must be aspirated.

Say someone has a warm knee. Even though it's ridiculously wrong, the hospitals will often call orthopedics, rheumatology, and infectious disease all the same time. It's crazy! I want to get there first so I can drain the knee and analyze the fluid. If I get there second, an orthopedist has already put the needle in the wrong place. Several times, I've had to reneedle the patient just to get the correct result. It's deeply frustrating.

But orthopedics brings in more money. People training to become orthopedic surgeons are often very financially motivated; orthopedics is listed as one of the highest paying subspecialties. At some point orthopedic surgeons decided there were too many spines to operate on, so they needed to do that too. But I don't believe they get the same training. I'm still a believer that spine surgery should be neurosurgical.

## Orthopedics Explained

When I consider what a good day looks like for me, I imagine on the schedule will be somebody complaining of finger pain, hand and wrist pain, knee pain, elbow pain, shoulder pain, or foot and ankle pain. The patient has already been to podiatry, orthopedics, and chiropractors—to everybody. But most patients going to orthopedics have no idea that they really belong in rheumatology. If I'm the only rheumatologist that can and will say that, so be it. It's the truth.

I'll say it again, even more clearly: anybody who is not seeing me and is seeing an orthopedic near me should see me instead.

This is where the specialty of rheumatology becomes more than just the ability to inject better and more precisely than the other guy. If I have a patient who is having toe pain, I look at the patient's toes. If I see a sausage toe, that person has psoriatic arthritis. I treat the patient with psoriatic medicine. I don't say it's infected and operate, which is a tragedy I've seen happen more times than I can count.

Or if I see white material extruding from under the toenail, I put it under the microscope and confirm whether it's gout, monosodium urate (MUS), or calcium hydroxyapatite. I don't say it's infected and call infectious disease. I don't take the patient to the operating room to debride it.

Worse yet, if there is a tissue specimen and you want to find gout, you need to know what fixative to use. It has to go in absolute alcohol because formaldehyde dissolves crystals. If you don't tell those who apply the fixative and you are not there, every specimen taken is sent in formaldehyde. The chance of finding the right thing is gone. How the hell am I the only one who knows that? I don't know—it's in the damn books. I learned it, and I remembered.

## Hand and Wrist

Common ailments I am an expert at treating (and have two patents for these needles) in the hands and wrists include arthritic knuckles, arthritic wrists—actually the first cmc-carpometacarpal joint—trigger fingers, and carpal tunnel syndrome. With trigger fingers, the tendon gets stuck, and the way to fix it is to stick a needle in the right place. If I do it right, there is success well in excess of 95 percent of the time for years or permanently. Two years later, the patient may come back for toe pain or back pain, and I'll say, "Weren't you here for trigger finger years ago?"

The patient will say, "Yeah, that went away after you injected it." It's a recurrent theme in my practice.

If the person instead goes to an orthopedic surgeon, the patient will get an injection that lasts for a week and then a surgery. When patients go to an orthopedic surgeon, always remember the surgeon is a hammer and the patients are seen as a nail.

Trigger fingers are common in alcoholics, diabetics, and others genetically predisposed. Why would you operate on these things if you can control their diabetes and give them one good injection? If the injection is done right, it works a high percentage of the time.

I see a lot of carpal tunnel syndrome. A person will say, "My hand is a little weak, and I have numbness in my thumb and the next two fingers. It's worse when I sleep and when I drive." When you sleep, you curl your wrist and compress the median nerve. When you drive, you extend your wrist and stretch the median nerve. The median nerve distribution is typically the first three and a half fingers. (The fingers are numbered one to five with the thumb being notated as one.) If the patient is between twenty and forty years old and is a normal individual who has a job, and if the history is unrevealing, I inject the person, who then gets better.

However, as a rheumatologist, I'm going to screen for pregnancy and thyroid disease. I want to be sure nothing else is going on. If the patient is an elderly man, I'm going to screen for amyloidosis. Your local orthopedic practitioner doesn't know these things because the doctor is only trained to operate on the carpal tunnel. The surgery for carpal tunnel is to remove the transverse ligament, which is the ligament or band on top of the median nerve. Often, the surgery doesn't work because the patient is diabetic and has an ischemic nerve, not an entrapment of the nerve. But now the ligament is gone, and guess what? The scar from the surgery now compresses the ischemic nerve. The patient goes back to the surgeon, and he or she gets a second surgery. The surgeon can't remove the ligament because it's already gone, so the scar tissue is removed instead, which just causes the scar to come back faster. Certain things are not meant to be removed; scar tissue is one of them.

I guarantee if the first surgery didn't work, the second one won't work either. It's insane! Patients who go through these operations later visit me and say, "You have to help me." I can put a needle in the area and if there is inflammation, it will help the patient, and *then* I can diagnose why inflammation is present. One can't just operate on people. Treat the underlying cause. It's like spraying gasoline on a fire to see if you can burn it out. Wouldn't it be smarter to get to the root of the fire before burning everything down?

The most common hand issue is osteoarthritis of the first carpometacarpal. I've gone all across the country injecting plastic surgeons, artists, bodybuilders, and dignitaries, and they all keep calling me if it ever comes back. They always tell me that they had it from the best hand surgeon in all of New York, the best hand surgeon at Scripps, from the best hand surgeon at Mayo, from the best hand surgeon at Hopkins. Well, I can't operate. But they don't inject like I do.

## The Art of Injecting

Injecting is a skill. It's one I didn't know I would need when I first found the field interesting.

In my rheumatology fellowship, I saw a patient who had lupus. Everything seemed okay except the patient's ankles hurt so bad that the pain prevented walking. I was perplexed. I said to my professor, "The patient is on such and such medicine and is tolerating the medicine, and the lungs are good, the muscles are good. The kidneys are good. But the person can't walk."

He said, "Well, did you think about an injection in the ankles?" I did not. "Go inject the ankles."

Before I went in the room, I'd read the book to see where I needed to put the needle. I then visited the patient, put the needle in the right place, and, *voila*, the person got up and walked away. The patient was fine.

I remember fielding a phone call once because the secretary had gone to the bathroom. It was a medical student calling because she had pain on the bottom of her foot. She thought she was calling orthopedics. I said, "This is rheumatology. Come here." She came right down. I examined her foot. She had a Morton neuroma—a nerve sheath tumor that's benign, usually between the second and third toes. If you inject it properly it just goes away. I know for a fact that ten years after I did that shot she was still better.

I'm injecting Depo-Medrol and lidocaine, with a lot of little tricks that are not taught. In the book, it says, for example, to use a .22-gauge needle for everything, and the length of the needle should be one-and-a-half inches. I have needles that are a half inch, one inch, one-and-a-half inches, three-and-a-half inches, six-and-a-half inches, seven-and-a-half inches, and nine inches. This is where people get unnecessarily scared. If you come at someone with a seven-and-a-half-inch needle, the patient will be petrified. I tell the patient, "No, the gauge of the needle is as small as it can be." If it's too small, it could break. But a three-and-a-half-inch needle at .25-gauge—that's beautiful! These patients come here all day long because nobody else can inject them. For orthopedic doctors to inject them, they'll either take them to the operating room or, worse, refer them to interventional radiology.

I do them all. The patients cannot be more grateful.

Take R. V. Turner, who is my general contractor, a great friend, and a patient of mine. He was about to go on disability. Doctors told him they would amputate his leg, they would replace his knee. He said, "Can you live on $500 a month? I can't. I'm not doing disability." Somehow, he came to me. He proudly brags that he waited for me for six hours on the first visit. But after he left, he never suffered again. He helped me lug a sofa upstairs after that! I thought we were both going to drop dead. But he did it, and he does it all the time. He's far from disabled after meeting me.

This is very common; everyone he met told him the shots don't work. Well, I went ahead and did it better. I put the needle in the right place.

## Foot and Ankle

Many common elements in the foot are rheumatological and should never be seen by anyone besides a rheumatologist. For somebody with heel pain and Achilles pain, for example, the heel pain is usually referable to the plantar fascia. It's not heel-spur pain. Many people have heel spurs and aren't aware; they don't hurt. It's the plantar fascia that gets inflamed. That is a feature of the group of diseases called spondyloarthropathy. In the classification of spondyloarthropathy are ankylosing spondylitis, psoriatic arthritis, Crohn disease-related arthritis, ulcerative colitis-related arthritis, sarcoidosis, and then rarities. It's one of those diseases. The good news is they're all treated very similarly and the treatment is usually effective. I may have to inject to get a patient out of pain and then treat the disease.

When I'm done with these people, they either have a diagnosis of a chronic disease with treatment or don't have a chronic disease and the conservative stuff worked.

## Knee Pain

I see many people with knee pain. A lot of them have arthritis but many don't. A lot have tendonitis or bursitis, neither of which is a surgical problem. The more common diagnoses would be arthritis, bursitis, and tendonitis, but we never want to miss a tumor—benign or malignant.

## Bursitis

Bursitis is inflammation of the bursa. Bursa are too numerous to count in the body, but some are known to get inflamed. Think of a bursa as something constitutionally like a jellyfish that occupies the space in the shape of a frisbee and the size of an oversized lifesaver mint. If you lie on your hip too long, a bursa can get inflamed. Women who are overweight inflame their pes anserine bursa, located about three inches below the medial portion of the knee. These people hurt walking on stairs. The bursa is exquisitely tender when inflamed. I inject it, and the pain goes away. Olecranon bursitis is a swollen golf ball on the elbow, which occurs with infection, gout, trauma, and more.

A lot of knee-pain patients have meniscal tears, most of which are not surgical problems. Three articles in the last ten years in the *New England Journal of Medicine*—if you can believe what it writes—indicate that meniscal surgery on an arthritic knee is neither necessary nor appropriate. It doesn't help anything. Those patients are still going to either need a knee replacement or get better with conservative steroid injections.

I can inject viscosupplements, which are genetically reprocessed hyaluronic acid—the major constituent of normal synovial fluid. This is routinely done, and the data is in favor of it. It's still covered by insurance.

However, Medicare decided you need a lot of physical therapy before they'll cover it. The truth, of course, is that the patients with arthritic knees are in too much pain in therapy, and nothing ends up happening because they quit therapy and are not allowed to get the shot. Or they have to pay out of pocket—yet another tragedy of our broken health-care system. Synvisc offers the unique pseudoseptic reaction; I try to avoid this product.

## Neck and Low Back

Most neck and low-back pain is muscular or mechanical. The most serious cause of back pain could be cancer, and we always treat the obvious and look for the most serious. In cervical or lumbar stenosis, where the nerves are involved, the neck is more important because if something happens to the nerves in your neck, you can become paraplegic.

Here's a little anatomy lesson: The brain and spinal cord are the same. The spinal cord in most people ends at the level of L1 or L2. Below L1 or L2 are nerve roots, not the actual spinal cord. The brain and spinal cord are referred to as upper motor neurons, and the peripheral nerves are referred to as lower motor neurons. If someone has a stroke, which is an upper motor neuron problem, you notice the person is spastic; they can't move their arm but it's spastic. If you were to cut a nerve root after it exits the spine, it becomes flaccid. Paralysis has two types: spastic and flaccid. With the flaccid paralysis, the reflexes go away, and with the spastic, the reflexes are abnormally brisk.

The tricky thing with the neck is that the spinal cord goes through it. A problem with a spinal cord is called a myelopathy. A problem with a nerve root leaving the spinal cord is called a radiculopathy. Cervical stenosis gives a myelopathy of the feet—the feet get spastic and clumsy because the stenosis is an upper motor neuron lesion to the feet, even though it's in the neck.

If a patient with a cervical stenosis has weakness in the hands with clumsy feet, check the neck. If cord compression exists, the person goes straight to the neurosurgeon. If the patient has stenosis without being in the danger zone, you send that person to pain management for an epidural injection. The orthopedic might send the patient to *that practitioner's* pain management, and who knows what may happen then. The patient could be sent to therapy and might end up paralyzed.

If the patient does not have a myelopathy, I can often inject the facet joints. The patient has arthritic spurs that can't be shrunk, but any inflammation around them is irritating. A course of high-dose oral steroids, a very strong muscle relaxer, and an anti-inflammatory medication will drastically help that patient.

Back during my training, I had a very interesting conversation with a neurosurgeon who was operating on a patient with lumbar spinal stenosis. The surgeon went in from the back, opened up the skin, and dissected down and removed bone and ligament that was causing pressure on the nerves. I said to him, "I thought the treatment for lumbar spinal stenosis was epidural injections."

He said, "Yeah, they work, but they don't last."

He was not wrong. But today, I get people who are seventy-five years old with high blood pressure, diabetes, heart attacks. They're not surgical candidates, but they want to walk. Although I don't do epidurals, I inject their facet joints. By injecting the proper joints, they go from being unable to stand and walk to having three or six months of freedom.

Years ago, I would do them every three months. Now, if they have Medicare, sorry. They can get two per year or one per year, depending on which region they live in. That's the politics of medicine—always looking out for everyone but the patient.

## Shoulder

Shoulder pain is extremely common, though I do not see much that I cannot inject and cure. What I can treat includes tendonitis of the rotator cuff and biceps, bursitis, and most types of arthritis. Most patients have one symptom in common: they cannot sleep on the affected shoulder due to pain.

If the joint is the problem, then the patient has an arthritic process. If I touch a painful tendon, the patient has tendonitis. If I touch a tender bursa that becomes painful, the patient has bursitis.

By watching the person move and looking for muscle atrophy, I can learn a lot. All patients with shoulder pain feel it at night because they lean on the painful or irritated shoulder, which wakes them up. Just by talking to a patient, I can assess the pain very quickly. While I talk to the person, I touch and see how the patient can move and which movements are restricted.

The rotator cuff or the biceps may get caught at the acromioclavicular joint, leading to fraying of the tendon. When it frays and then heals and calcifies, one can get calcific tendonitis. You don't want to remove the calcium because it's going to grow back. You don't want to do anything. The patient needs to avoid tears if possible, but tears don't usually require surgery. The tear that does is the complete tear. The rotator cuff has four muscles. If one is damaged, three others are left. The patient needs to work on strengthening the other three. All of these areas are amenable to injections. The one that is the least amenable to injections happens to be tennis elbow, which is tendonitis of the lateral epicondyle, on the outside of the elbow.

## Arthritis

To the lay population, there is the good kind of arthritis and the bad kind. The good kind is osteoarthritis. That's the noninflammatory kind, although research shows that inflammation really is a component. The bad kind is the inflammatory arthritis. The first thing is to identify inflammation, swelling, morning stiffness, redness, tenderness, warmth, and so on. If there is inflammation—remember my beautiful charts—is it connective tissue disease, such as rheumatoid arthritis, lupus, Sjogren syndrome, scleroderma, or myositis?

Is the problem an infection, such as Lyme, infectious endocarditis, hepatitis B, hepatitis C, HIV, syphilis, or gonorrhea? Gonorrhea still remains the most common cause of monoarthritis of the knee in young women. And do not forget travel hepatitis A, zika, or chikungunya.

Then, consider spondyloarthropathy, including ankylosing spondylitis, psoriatic arthritis, Crohn colitis, ulcerative colitis, sarcoidosis. The next category consists of crystals named monosodium urate (gout), calcium pyrophosphate (pseudogout). FYI: pseudogout is calcium pyrophosphate deposition disease, basic calcium phosphate (hydroxyapatite), and so on.

Another category, termed fibrocartilaginous diseases, is somewhat exclusive to a newly defined condition, IgG4-related disease.

Arthritis refers to inflamed or painful joints. Is the joint inflamed? Or is it just painful?

Everyone throws around the acronym DJD, which stands for degenerative joint disease. It is used incorrectly in place of osteoarthritis. A purist who cares about the terminology can't use the acronym DJD without excluding all the other secondary forms of osteoarthritis. Incorrect usage of *degenerative joint disease* leads to incorrect diagnosis and treatment.

People who use terminology incorrectly aren't trained. A lot of the people in this field don't care. Radiologists often point out something that's irrelevant and overlook something that isn't. Every day people tell me, "I've been to everybody, and nobody can help me."

I ask why they didn't come to me sooner.

"I never heard about you until I asked my friends."

I say, "If your doctor didn't refer you, the doctor isn't good for you, because how can the doctor not know me if I've been here for thirty years?"

I wish I knew the answer to this question. To be fair, I think my brazen New York personality and outspokenness are not acceptable to a lot of people. I merely say I'm a very strong patient advocate, and I advocate for good medicine, not bad. I cannot tell you how many of my fellow rheumatologists have been sued and I have been asked to be an expert witness. I would never attack them; anybody can make a legitimate error. Let's be honest—jealousy is a tremendous factor. Beyond that, who knows?

If a patient has hip and back pain and can't cross the legs, the back pain is somehow referred from the hips. I have to decipher what the patient means when saying something hurts. That means arthritis if it's in the front, bursitis if it's on the side, or related to the spine if it's in the back. But without the proper diagnosis, there is no hope of getting the proper treatment. Without a rheumatologist, they'll all end up in surgery.

## Who Should See an Orthopedic?

To summarize this chapter: for all of these things, people often end up in orthopedics, they end up with surgery which doesn't fix the problem and often causes more problems. Proper diagnosis is overlooked. In a perfect world, anybody who goes to the emergency room, urgent care, or the family doctor and complains of pain should be sent to a good rheumatologist first. If you are reading this you very well may need joint surgery, reconstruction, or replacement. Consider an opinion from a rheumatologist as there is no motivation for surgery. Should you need the surgery there are many excellent well-trained orthopedic surgeons available to help you.

I've discovered and written about gout in the artificial joint. The reason I wrote the paper is orthopedics were telling people it's not possible. When people say, "I was told I can't have it more than once a year," I explain to them that it's like washing your underwear in bleach. You can't do that every day because you'll destroy the underwear. But you could still have underwear for five years if you just wash it properly. (Patients are told they cannot get gout in an artificial joint which is false. Patients are told they cannot have corticosteroid injections into a joint more than a certain number of times. This has some truth. The reality is if you are injecting a joint too often, it really says the joint injections are not working for that problem.)

All of which is not to say good orthopedic surgeons don't have a role. A really good surgeon can literally save somebody's hand. If a zookeeper gets bitten by a lion and the tendons are severed, the zookeeper needs a very skilled orthopedic surgeon to sew them back together. The orthopedic surgeon, though, would probably refer the zookeeper to a plastic surgeon because the orthopedic surgeon can make more money operating on spines. There are individuals who for various reasons simply cannot have joint injections. An example would be those with osteonecrosis or dead bone. These patients, if in pain, must have knee replacement if physical therapy and pain relievers do not work. Corticosteroid injections will worsen this condition.

The rheumatologist is the most important doctor you can have. The rheumatologist is an internal medicine specialist and an orthopedic specialist combined. We diagnose and treat complicated internal medicine, which are the really interesting diseases, and all joint and bone diseases. We're the ones who know all the diseases and the patterns of joint involvement. We know how to make the diagnosis. Rheumatologists know where to look to put it all together. We're the ones who say, "No, you don't have six problems when your eyes hurt or are red, your belly hurts, you have fevers and sweats, and you have joint pain. That's adult-onset Still disease [or Behcet's disease or some crazy arthritic condition]."

Non-rheumatologists have no clue. There could be pus coming out of all the joints, and they don't know the difference between pus and gout. It never comes to me like it should.

Why? Ignorance—plus, orthopedic doctors are present in the hospital, showing their face.

Say a patient is sent to ortho for epidural and osteoarthritis. Stop right there. The patient has osteoarthritis? Why wouldn't that person go to an arthritis specialist? Why would he or she go to a bone surgeon?

The rheumatologist is the only expert on arthritis, but arthritis patients get to a rheumatologist a small percent of the time. Arthritis is incredibly common.

A rheumatologist is a medical specialist trained in nonsurgical orthopedics or, in other words, bone and joint diseases, not bone and joint injuries—at least not usually. Exceptions such as a posttraumatic gout attack would be a situation for a rheumatologist, not an orthopedic surgeon. The emergency room is programmed to call orthopedics and unfortunately the patient ends up with the incorrect care. For every disease an orthopedic surgeon treats—arthritic joints or lower back, hands or wrists carpal tunnel, foot problems, plantar fascia, Achilles tendon—the patients all need a rheumatologist. A rheumatologist is not trained in surgery and an orthopedic surgeon is not trained in diagnosing and treating inflamed painful joints. They operate, which wastes time and money, causes pain and suffering, and typically only makes the problem worse.

To finish, I'll say it once more. To anybody seeing an orthopedist for joint pain, I would advise seeing a rheumatologist who is highly skilled at injecting joints and tendons. To anyone who can, I recommend seeing me!

# ABOUT THE AUTHOR

Dr. Stephen Soloway is known within the medical community as a medical detective and will proudly announce, "If I can't fix you, I will get someone who can." His vast experience is second to none.

He is board certified in internal medicine since 1991, and rheumatology since 1993, and recertified four times since, with specialized certificates in osteoporosis. Dr. Soloway is chairman of the Department of Rheumatology Division of Internal Medicine Inspira Health Network. His credentials also include clinical associate professor at Rowan University School of Osteopathic Medicine, adjunct clinical associate professor at Drexel University College of Medicine, Castle Connolly American's Top Doctor, and *Philadelphia* magazine and *Inside Jersey* magazine Top Doctor. He is regarded as a regional and national leader in rheumatologic care. His main office is in southern New Jersey with easy access to Philadelphia, Atlantic City, Delaware, Philadelphia, New York City, and the world.

Dr. Soloway proudly notes that he was placed on this earth to help people, and dedicated his life to the diagnosis and treatment of peers, patients, dignitaries, world leaders, and professional athletes, to name a few. He's had patients visit him from fifty countries and nearly one hundred US cities. He is involved in arthritis, gout, and osteoporosis treatment and has a passion for joint injections. Currently, he has nine patents approved or pending—in the US and abroad—related to needles and injection techniques that he has perfected over his career. His patents pave the way for nonsurgical treatment of trigger finger, carpal tunnel, and arthritic wrist. Amongst his publications, he is most proud of the discovery of gout and pseudogout in artificial joints, and a rare disease article on Bechet's disease featured in the *New England Journal of Medicine*.

Through his previous book, *Bad Medicine: The Horrors of American Healthcare*, and his popular YouTube channel, Dr. Soloway has taught tens of thousands of people how to advocate for themselves, fight against a broken system, and win against Big Pharma, Big Insurance, and Big Government.

Dr. Soloway has a presidential appointment and is the president of the Israel Heritage Foundation.

Dr. Soloway enjoys giving back to the community through charity and by teaching patients and doctors. He lives in southern New Jersey.

# ACKNOWLEDGMENTS

Without the unwavering support and unconditional love bestowed upon me by my amazing late parents, Frances and Warren, there would be no book. "Go where your life will be the best. We will follow you there."

My children, Alyxandra, MD, and Jacob: I instill strong values and teach you the virtue of why daddy comes home late too often.

Without these men, I would not have the tools to be in my own shoes: M. Anthony Albornoz, MD, Bruce Hoffman, MD, H. R. Schumacher, Jr., MD, Lawrence Leventhal, MD.

To my best friends and coworkers, your timeless devotion can't be measured: David Weksel, Robert Feferman, MD, Kurt Henry, MD (DK Star Productions); Debra Richards, CEO; Denise Lister, CMA; Dana Solomon, CMA; Audrey Rubano, NP (proof I am a Rheum fellowship), Julia Tillman; Tim Lieske, Rosanne pastor (deceased).

And Martin Koslin (love you Uncle Martin). Plus Ariel and Sarah!

To those nurses and physician assistants that I have trained and who have gone into rheumatology. They have taught me as much as I have taught them:

- Audrey Rubano
- Cicily Jeannette
- Timyra Lister
- Laurie Nichols
- Lyndy Tanimae
- Elaine Lange
- Marianne Gibbons (deceased)
- Kelly Cervini

- Matt Arkebauer, DO
- Tyler and Alexandria Chin, in memory of Marven Chin

And the tens of thousands of appreciative patients.